318

A CHUBBY CHICK'S TALE
OF WEIGHT LOSS SURGERY

Jessyca Mathews

authorHOUSE®

AuthorHouse™
1663 Liberty Drive
Bloomington, IN 47403
www.authorhouse.com
Phone: 1 (800) 839-8640

Published by AuthorHouse   03/08/2016

ISBN: 978-1-5049-8435-5 (sc)
ISBN: 978-1-5049-8436-2 (e)

CONTENTS

Preface-May 2015 1

Making the Decision 15

Fat Flashback-My Slogan 18

Taking My First Step 21

And Here's a Bottle of Water 24

Sharing the News 29

The Family 34

Jumping through Hoops 38

Fat Flashback-Red Light Special with RKB 46

Starvation 53

Surgery Day 59

Pain and Pamela... 64

Keep on Loving You! 70

Did My Stomach Just Growl? 75

Fat Flashback High School Note Writing 78

Wasting Away 82

The Social Network... 87

Time for a Tightening... 89

Real Temptation 96

The Emotional, the Hormonal, and the Acne 102

Back to Work... 107

Fat Flashback-I Break Things… 112

Fitness.. 115

Fab Flashback-Getting People's Attention 121

Fat Flashback-Swimsuit Terror... 131

The Beginnings of Failure 135

Food Rejection 148

Five Years to the Day 151

Acknowledgements 159

About the Author 161

CONTENTS

Dedication:
To those who want a better life-
Stop waiting.
The time is now.

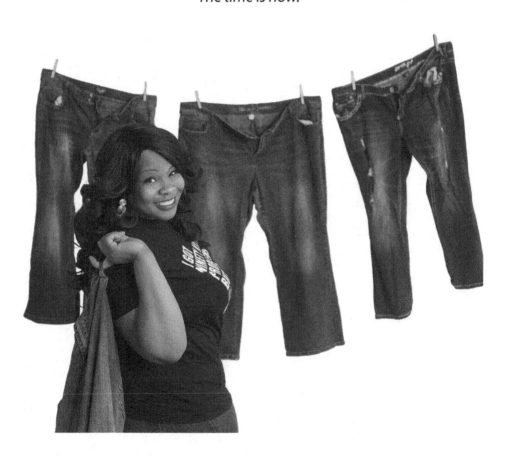

PREFACE-MAY 2015

"Congrats, Coach! Great win out there today! Tell Bill that I got you. We are going out to celebrate!"

"Celebrate? Now?" My voice quivered after hearing the declaration.

"Ummm, Coach. I don't know if that is a good..."

We were strolling side by side on a freshly cut soccer field. The sounds of jubilation from the players rang through the pollen-filled air, and parents were rushing to their children with glee. On an unusually warm May afternoon, we had a shutout. Our first win. Today was a perfect day. That is until I had to think about Coach Damiekco's comment.

I bit my lip. My mind was whirling with the right escape plan. I needed a valid excuse of why we should not go out for a festive meal.

No, we can't hang out. I have to go grade papers. I could check my phone and say that my family needed me.

I...

I needed...

I needed an escape.

Before I could even open my mouth to blubber out a lame reason, he cut me off. I didn't even get a chance to muster up a sentence.

"Girl, hurry up and get your stuff together. I'm driving. I'm feeding you. We can leave as soon as the girls are all gone."

I had spent so much energy on having a keen focus during the match and was joyous when the final whistle blew to signify victory, but the idea of going out to dinner suddenly made the palms of my hands begin to sweat. My worry was I would have to eat in front of a new person.

He would see how I have to eat.

He would have questions.

I would have to tell him my story.

My new JV coach, Damiekco, was probably the most open person that I have ever met. We had just met three months before the season started, but there came a time that he was quite expressive with me about his life and what made him into the charismatic man that he is. There were private conversations after away games when we sat on the school bench located near the gym's entrance. He had no issue with baring his soul on his upbringing, his choices, and his vision for his future. I admired his strength and openness.

Damiekco was not the problem in going out to eat. I could understand why many people would jump to that conclusion. From the outside looking in, he was near perfect: motivated, funny, loved children, and as he often declared to the players, he was "cute." He was the person that I found to be quite entertaining with his tales and always made me comfortable. When he talked, I listened. I giggled, frowned, and smiled while listening to his narration, but I hadn't shared much of my life. And now, the two of us were going out to eat. The food was what made me nervous, not the man.

I wasn't ready.

I didn't know if I could bring myself to tell him why I had to eat differently than most people. The necessity of sharing about my surgery and its effects hadn't yet played a role in our conversations up to this moment. The topic of my eating rituals would lead to questions followed by my answers that usually made people cringe. I didn't want him to question my decision in why I made such a strange choice for my life, or to chastise me for taking such a dangerous route to a new path. But now, I was about to go out to dinner with him. There was no avoiding this issue. If I went out to have a meal with him, this would open up a conversation that was always awkward to have.

"Coach, I'm going to need you to get your life together and get going so we can eat. Stop staring into space and let's get these girls out of here. I'm starving!"

I had gone from walking in stride with him to falling far behind. I was trapped in an analytical haze on this issue and had suddenly become petrified in the middle of our soccer field. I frantically raced to catch up with him, feeling foolish that I had been daydreaming of a way to escape. While rushing to catch up with him, I looked to the sky in search for a sign of what I should do. Should I just say "no" to his idea? Am I too sensitive on the topic? The clouds didn't give me an answer. The sun just kept on shining. There was no way out.

After packing up game balls, placing corner flags in the shaded area of the storage unit, locking the gate, and waving to the last girl to be picked up by her parent, I went to my best friend, Bill, who was my timekeeper for games.

I needed for my friend to be an excuse. Forcing him to listen to me would, at least, give me an opportunity to run. Maybe I would find a way to convince myself to hop in the car with him and not go out and share an aspect of my life with someone new.

While standing in front of Bill, my voice began to stammer.

"Yeah. Ummm, you go ahead home. I'm going to catch a ride with Damiekco. He wants to feed me."

He raised his eyebrows and blinked inquisitively at me. He went to question me but stopped. I didn't need to tell him my worries. In many ways, we shared a brain, and he knew that I had an issue with eating in front of new people. Bill reached out for my soccer bag. He wouldn't have any part in this situation. I saw the corners of his lips curl upward, and his head gave a gentle nod.

"Bill, I..."

He wouldn't hear my complaints. As quick as a flash, Bill had unlocked the car door and hopped inside. Before closing the driver's side door, he yelled out only four words.

"You two have fun."

He left me there, standing in an aggravated state. I guess he thought he was doing what was best for me, although I wanted to punch the side of his jaw. Bill was forcing me to deal with my food issues. I secretly stuck up my middle finger at him as he zoomed away, leaving me standing there to deal with my current inner conflict.

The sound of gravel crunched with the soles of shoes coming up behind me. Damiekco approached bearing his usual comforting grin, and just said, "You ready to go, Coach?"

I couldn't get out of it.

A short moment later, I found myself guided toward a massive, American-made truck. Being of short stature, I had to struggle with stepping up into this monstrosity. I gripped the handle, pulled myself onto the vehicle step and plopped down in the passenger seat. My hand fiddled around to find the seat belt, and I tried to control the fearful thoughts that were racing in my mind.

Damiekco, filled with enormous energy, slipped into the truck with ease. The truck style didn't surprise me. It was flashy, filled with reminders of his love for the game of soccer and his daughter, and screamed for observers to notice its beauty. It was cold black and was a pure reflection of him. There was a hum as he turned the ignition, a series of clicks from changing from park to drive, and then we began our ride.

"Since you are the big winner for today, I'm gonna let you THINK that you are special, Coach."

I cut my eyes over in his direction, and he once again flashed a huge grin. Comments of this style were his way of treating you kindly and picking on you at the same time. I looked away and shook my head slowly at his antics.

"I'm buying whatever you want. Choose where you want to eat and I'm paying for it. You have to be starving," Damiekco claimed.

He was right.

I was starving.

It had been a long day: six hours in the classroom and multiple hours out on the field can make a girl hungry. My lunchtime was scheduled too early for my medical condition. Most people are just having breakfast at 10:45, but I was supposed to be having the second meal of the day. Rarely did a full lunch period happen for me. Most times, there was a senior coming in either begging for extra credit, crying due to confusions about the world, or asking the umpteenth time if they were passing the class. If I were lucky, I would get 15 minutes to myself to chew a small part of my sandwich. I could always count on never completing my meal due to how I have to eat. There is always too much to do.

So yes, I was starving. But hearing him say that I could pick where to eat made me lose part of my appetite. All I could do was bite my lip slightly again and listen to him while he drove away from the school.

I was able to make small conversation on the road and finally chose a restaurant for us to visit. Moments later, we were there. I found myself hopping out the truck. Damiekco raced in front of me to open the door in a gentleman-like fashion. My legs, thick with dread, clunked up to the door, and I stepped inside.

Seating was available right away when we entered the restaurant. There were a limited number of people scattered at booths and tables, and one middle-aged man found semi-slumped at the bar with a half empty glass of alcohol resting in his hands. We sat in a booth located in the far left corner, near televisions filled with sporting events. There was classic satellite radio music humming from the restaurant's speakers. After being seated, a pleasant hostess supplied us with menus. She rambled off the specials that were on the tap and asked us what beverages we wanted to have.

"I'll just have water, thank you," was my reply.

"Really, Coach? Water? I'm paying for your meal, and you want to get some water?"

So, it begins. I didn't want to tell him I no longer could drink pop.

"I'm good with just water, Coach. I just finished coaching and just need to recharge. It's not a diss on you and your money you're itching to burn up on me."

We both giggle and he decides that he will just have water, too. Both of us are relaxed and begin to scan our menus.

I have to make my selection carefully. I look over the menu and analyze it like I have had to do for almost five years. I start going down my mental checklist:

No, you can't get a burger. You haven't had one in forever. It's not your friend. You don't want to get sick.

No, don't get that sandwich. The bread is thick, and it will just come right back out as soon as you start to eat it. The last thing you want to do is throw up on your new JV coach. Plus, he would never let that one go.

No, steak. Too expensive, even with him saying get what you want. Plus, it doesn't break down well either.

No, don't get just an appetizer. He will never let you just get an app. I don't want to offend him.

Not that.

Or that.

Never that...

Before, I just ate what I wanted. I didn't have to go through and examine a menu like an ameba under a microscope. I just ate. Not anymore. I had to be careful.

"Have you decided what you would like to have?" The tall male server had appeared, smiling from ear to ear. His long, tan fingers were gripping a pencil and order pad, and he was waiting for me. Damiekco had already ordered his burger and fries, and he too was waiting for my reply.

"Oh, yes. I need this sandwich but do not put on the tomato or the barbecue sauce. Oh, and light lettuce if it's not too much to ask. Does it come with anything other than fries?"

After hearing a complicated answer from our server, I decided that I didn't want to make my meal seem like a complete train wreck. I took the fries instead of picking a different side dish and asked for the condiments on the side for me to dip my food. The server repeated my order and smiled as if it wasn't a chore to make it the way that I wanted it. He stated that he would be back with our meals as soon as possible.

When I looked across the table, I found Damiekco looking over inquisitively. I quietly shuttered and fumbled with my napkin under the table. My skin was on pins and needles, and I couldn't avoid his glare. I wanted something to break the stare down from across the table. Glasses clinked in the back from the restaurant's staff. Finally, he spoke.

"Coach?" Damiekco uttered.

I sighed, preparing for the inquisition.

"Yes, Coach?" I murmured.

"Do you think our server is gay? Because I think that he is. I don't have a problem with it, but I have to know if my gay guess is right," he jokingly whispered.

I tilted my head down into my chest and started to chuckle. I thought he was going to question my order, but he was more fascinated by the choice of mate of our waiter. We both started giggling at his comment, and we both were ready to talk to one another in a friendly tone once again.

We chatted, and my body began to relax. He shared more stories of his life, and I started to see why he was such a fascinating person. He shared things that most would keep hidden from the world, and I told him that I appreciated him being so open. This dinner was the first time that we had thought of one another as friends instead of co-workers. As soon as I felt the most comfortable with him, the slender, could-be-gay server appeared with our food. The time was now. He would have to notice.

After receiving my plate, I laid eyes on my food. There was a part of me that thought that if I quickly began my ritual, maybe he wouldn't notice. It had been such an enjoyable 20 minutes, but I knew that things were about to change. Panic started to set in once again. I had to act. It's time to eat.

Quickly, I unwrapped my silverware, and I began my food methodology:

A glass of water pushed to the far side of the table, almost hidden.

You can't eat and drink at the same time-It's there in case of emergency only.

A dab of ketchup on the corner of the plate. Too much, too many calories.

Grab the knife. Take a deep breath. You know what you have to do.

Cut the sandwich in half.

Cut the halves into quarters for baby portions.

Take half the fries and push them far to the side of the plate.

You won't be eating all of those.

Put a dab of mustard near the ketchup, just enough to enjoy.

Inspect the sandwich for anything that would be difficult to digest.

Pray over your food.

Pray that it stays down.

When I finished, I picked up the tiny piece of sandwich and began to chew. My food methodology continues without me looking at him:

Chew 15 times.

Chew 10 more times.

If not completely turned into mush, chew an additional 5-10 times.

Swallow but don't drink the water.

I glanced up. A pair of chocolate eyes was looking at me. His burger was in his hands, but he paused his position to examine how I was eating. He was chewing furiously on his burger, but he didn't stop watching me. The aroma of the grilled beef that he was holding up in the air was making me jealous. I wanted his meal. I wanted that burger.

"What gives, Coach? Why did you do that to your sandwich?"

The moment was now. Again, I crossed my hands under the table. The napkin began to become wadded up in my fingers.

"What do you mean, Damiekco?"

My voice wobbled. There was no way that my statement would make him not ask what was going on. I knew he would be persistent.

His voice level increased with forceful intrigue.

"Don't play like you didn't understand me, woman. What's the deal?"

He placed his burger down on his plate and leaned backward in his seat. His attention was solely on me. It was time for me to explain myself. Ready or not, I was in the situation in which I had to share what I do with food.

I took my hands out from hiding, placed the torn napkin on the table top, and pushed my plate slightly aside before I began to share my story.

"Well, Coach. Almost five years ago, I kind of had this surgery."

His posture changed, and he leaned forward with interest. It was the first thing that I had been willing to share with him, and he looked at me filled with wonder and attentiveness. Finally, he had cracked my shell. He would learn something about me.

"What kind of surgery?"

"Bariatric surgery. I had this procedure called gastric banding done."

He tilted his head.

"Did it hurt?"

"Yes, very much so for the first couple weeks. Every once in a while, I have a terrible band day, but for the most part, it's been normal."

I gave him a summary of the surgery, just enough to make sure that he wouldn't lose his appetite. He continued to eat his meal but paid attention to my tale, asking small questions of curiosity. Thing went easy until I shared how much I could eat.

"See, Damiekco, I have to cut my food up into small bites so that it goes down smoothly. The smaller, the better for my stomach. And I have to chew at least 25 times, take a break, and then eat some more. I appreciate you buying me the meal, but I'm only getting through about half of this," I advised.

His eyes grew large at the statement, and he dipped the remainder of his fries into a glob of ketchup. He chewed quickly, swallowed hard, and parted his lips with more questions.

"Only half of this? You didn't even order that much! How much can you eat?"

"About a cup and a half at a time," I reported.

"Oh HELL NAW!" Damiekco exclaimed. We both look around to see if others heard his borderline profanity. No one reacted, and both of us laughed. I reached over and took another piece of my sandwich and started to nibble. Damiekco continued.

"You survive on eating that little amount of food? Damn, I couldn't make it. I would be tooooo hungry."

After finishing the tiny morsel of my meal, I replied.

"You get used to it. The band won't let you go passed that amount. That's the whole purpose of getting it done. It regulates me, and I don't mind anymore."

"What happens if you keep eating?" he asked.

"Then I throw up on you," I replied.

He jerked back in disgust.

"Oh. Yeah, let's stick to the plan. Never that. Not on me."

Both of us laughed again.

Damiekco then asked me something that one ever asked me before.

"Does it scare you to talk about it?"

I paused and thought back on the process that I went through to become the woman I was sitting at the table. There was pain, there was stress, but most of all, there was success. I was healthier. I was stronger, but I still had issues as simple as eating in front of people. I was winning, but I hadn't completed the race. With it all, there were times that I was still scared and needed a reminder that with each battle I would become stronger.

"Sometimes. Sometimes it does scare me to talk about it. Especially with new people. Oddly, I've written down what has happened to me from the surgery, but I stumble with being judged by others. Does that make sense?"

His eyes squinted as if he was in deep thought, and he leaned forward so that he could talk just loud enough so that the two of us could hear it.

"Coach. You can share things with me. You don't have to be scared. I got you."

At that moment, he gave me what I needed. I didn't need to be afraid to tell people who I was and what I have become. After almost five years of living with the band writing down events that have changed my life, I was ready to share my story.

_____

MAKING THE DECISION

Hefty. Thick. Chunky. These were some of the descriptive words that friends and family tried used to cover up the obvious weight problem I had for almost three decades of my life. For a long time, I identified with these words.

I was "hefty" when I was starting the fifth grade. This was the first time I noticed that my face was rounder than all my skinny girlfriends. At eleven years old, I started to notice my hips were growing larger and my chest was starting to poke out from underneath my classic 80's themed t-shirts. I noticed that the seams were clinging on to dear life to keep my body covered with every pair of jeans I slipped on for school. My mom blamed it on hormones, and stressed that I was just taking the steps to "becoming a real woman." I was developing faster than everyone else, and everything would be alright according to Mom, but I knew it was the beginning of the stares and the insults from the boy classmates. This would be the starting place of my weight battles for years to come.

I moved up to "thick" when I got into middle and high school. I was a "solid" girl, one who played three sports and was voted the "Most Athletic" in the Class of '95 by my peers, but I still struggled to find a uniform that didn't fit snuggly around my ever growing hips and broad shoulders. I was the girl who the night before a big game had to soak her game day gear in water, and then tug on the sleeves of the jersey and the waistband of my shorts as if I were blessed with super human strength just to make each piece of my uniform fit a little looser.

"Chunky" came with adulthood, and many medical mishaps took over my body with a vengeance. Heavier pounds arrived in college when I started to have female issues. First, the back pain and the need for pain killers, then the cysts, the birth control pills with dangerous side effects soon followed. Then the blot clot came. The tumors were next. Each stage added 10 pounds here, 15 there, until I had a fear of standing on the scales in all four of my doctor's offices.

"Hefty", "thick" and "chunky" were the words growing up. By the time I reached my 30's, I was just plain ol' fat.

It was November 2nd when I reached this conclusion, while standing in my bathroom, staring at my then warped, naked, disfigured body in a long, elegant mirror. The rolls that had taken over my midsection told me I was fat. The skin flapping from my upper arms that gave the appearance of parts of the local car wash let me know I was fat. The stretch marks expressway that traveled down my chest, my back, and my tan thighs let me know I was fat.

The cute little names from childhood, my teen years, and my early 20s to cover up my excessive weight didn't change the obvious that I reached by age 33. The pep talks of the past that I was, "Fine the way I was" didn't change a damn thing. All the diets, the obsessive working out, the cutting out bad foods hadn't changed anything. I was fat.

I remember turning around and looking at every dimension of my body on that day. The deep dimples behind my knees that sunk into my skin, the place where my waist use to be was round with pudgy skin, and the birthmark that used to be on the upper portion of my right glut that had slowly crept down at least two inches. I took three small steps forward and leaned in to frown at the grotesque figure starting at me in the mirror.

Finally, with complete detestation and disgruntlement, I stopped examining my defaulted figure and looked at the most important part of my body. I took a long, deep look into my brown almond-shaped eyes. They were so troubled, so tormented, and more importantly, so unhealthy.

"You need to change. Stop waiting. You need to change," is all I could muster up to say quietly to myself, as a soft, simple tear fell down my round face.

FAT FLASHBACK-MY SLOGAN

When I was 10, my grandmother, my brother, Chris, sister, Angi, and I went out for the annual Kalamazoo summer shopping trip. It was standard procedure that we spent at least two weeks of our summer vacation in Kalamazoo with my grandparents when we were young, which meant my grandmother would take us shopping for school clothes. I don't recall the specific store, but for some reason they had buttons for sale. My grandmother said we could each buy a button since they were a dollar a piece (she wouldn't buy anything that wasn't on sale). The buttons were placed in a large, blue bin at the end of the school supply aisle, which was brilliant strategic placement for impulse buyers like my grandmother. My siblings and I ran over to the bin, and we began to rummage through the collection, looking for a cool button that represented us to put on our backpacks for the first day of school. Chris found a button about being smart.

My brother, who is two years younger than I, is probably the smartest person I know. He can read a map like an old prospector when we traveled, and could babble off history and music facts way before the Internet had provided easy answers for us. Everyone in the family knew he was the quickest to pick up on small observations of people, places, and things, so it was only natural that he brags about his intelligence with a shiny, new button.

Angi, is the cute one. She has always been gorgeous, even as a baby people would coo over her radiance. She was the cheerleader in school; the one everyone knew and was voted to Top 10 for homecoming princess. Even before Angi had boys falling to her feet in high school, she was the doll in kindergarten, and she was about to take on the first grade after this summer. It was only fitting that Angi's button had to deal with her being a beautiful princess. The world already knew this, but the button would give her a stamp of approval. Especially with a button with a pretty, white crown.

I was struggling to find a button. There were no tomboy buttons about whooping the boys' asses in dodge ball in gym class. There were no "middle of the road beauty" buttons, no "I am smart, but not as smart as my brother" buttons. One after another I picked up a button and then tossed it to the side. Searching through the pile of buttons was torture, especially for an elementary girl who was entering the fifth grade. I had to find one for the first day of school for my backpack!

My grandmother sensed I needed assistance and began to dig. She raced through the buttons on the right side of the bin, while I feverishly dug on the left for my own personal slogan to declare my self-importance. Suddenly my grandmother exclaimed, "Mmmmhmmmm! Jessy, what about this one? It's hilarious!"

I was excited; finally, I too, would have a badge of honor to wear to Dye Elementary, proclaiming my greatness! I couldn't wait to read what it said, and how the world would see me, especially if it was funny. Many had said that they enjoyed my sense of humor. Rather rudely, I pushed my siblings out of the way, and I reached over the shopping cart, eagerly waiting to see my button. My declaration!

It was a bright pink button with white, cloud-like shaped writing on it. I read the statement on the button and a knot suddenly appeared in my stomach.

"I'm not fat, I'm fluffy."

I looked down at the button again, and then down at my body. At 10, I already had a chest and was wearing a big girl bra. My hips spread out on both sides, and I definitely didn't look like girls in the teen magazines that I read. I was bigger than everyone else, in every way.

My grandmother meant no harm, and the button was funny, but it didn't change how I felt. I felt my cheeks grow hot with embarrassment, and I heard my brother and sister giggle at what it said. The button was just a joke about people's physical status. Or was my body the bigger joke?

I wanted to go home…

TAKING MY FIRST STEP

Gastric Banding (or GB as I like to call it) commercials caught my attention years before I started my journey. Actually, I thought about getting "GBed" after seeing commercials three years before I started the process, but I wasn't completely ready mentally. I remember I went and spoke to my family doctor three years before actually having the surgery and he said "absolutely not" to give me medical clearance. It was his belief that if I kept exercising and sticking to my diet of "no pop and watching my carbs" I could magically lose 100 pounds. After hearing him say "No" to the idea, I went to my parents. My mother thought it was a good idea, but my father was completely against it. He had known someone who had lost their life in another style of bariatric surgery, and wasn't too keen on my being a guinea pig for some new procedure. So, I gave up on the idea, and sunk back into my fatness.

The first piece of advice that I can give is don't make the decision to have gastric banding solely on what others say. Ask others' opinions, but the choice is completely up to you, and only you! When you are ready to take the plunge, go 100% toward your goal, or you will never have it done and start your new life. Don't do it because you are trying to look good for a man, don't do it because other people where you work do it, and don't do it thinking it will make everything all better. You have to be mentally, spiritually, and physically ready, and when you are ready, do it!

I wasn't ready in 2007 because I let other people's views control my choices. I let my doctor tell me what was right for me, and I let my family say what was right for me. I should've let ME say what was right for ME!

Years passed and I made excuses. School made it so I couldn't do it during nine months of the year. Coaching made it so I couldn't do it four months of the year. I ran a semi-professional football team during the summer, so that time wasn't the right time to do it. School and work filled my calendar, and I couldn't care for myself. I couldn't take time for me to get better.

As time passed I gained more pounds on my frame and became unhealthier. I had fast food during the sports seasons. There was stressful candy popping during exam week with me being a teacher. I was too tired to cook a healthy dinner, and sometimes I didn't eat dinner at all. I believed that this lifestyle would never catch up to me, but slowly and surely, my unhealthy lifestyle took over, and I didn't know how to control what was happening to me.

At one point I did make a change for the better, and I got into exercising and began to eat healthier. I made healthy choice commitments and gave up unnecessary calories. I gave up candy popping and took away wasteful calories. One major obstacle that I conquered was an addiction to pop. I became hooked in college, and didn't realize the intake of sugar I was putting into my body until I read a news article about the effects on the human immune system. I started drinking more water, eating more salads, taking walks in the evening, and I began to see progress. After my rebirth into health consciousness, I lost almost 30 pounds and felt great about my accomplishment, but even with the healthier life, I gain it all back plus another five. It was beyond frustrating, and I almost gave up. After having the bathroom mirror moment, I knew that enough was enough. I would make the change to make myself healthier. So, I went back to that same informational website, and began my real "GB" journey for my goal of better health.

I went to my search engine, and began the steps toward a better life. The first site that I was directed to was lapband.com, and I began to read. The website was overwhelming! There was so much information that I needed to shift through. There was a listing of doctors, their awards, accreditation and degrees, and reviews of their performance. There were videos explaining the procedure, and success stories of those who dared to take the plunge into bariatric surgery. My heart raced at the possibility to get healthy, to become the person that I knew had been inside of me for so long. The inner me could play soccer again, and run on a treadmill without getting completely winded. She could walk in a mall without getting dirty looks and snickers from children passing by. The inner self could stand on a scale without getting nauseous and shaking with fear, and she could be proud of her looks, her health, and could hold her head high.

In the upper right hand corner there was a button labeled "Attend a Free Seminar." I felt like it had a blessed glow, pouring its thinner and healthier grace out upon me. I reached for my mouse, and clicked the button to set a date. There was free seminar at a bariatric center in December.

AND HERE'S A BOTTLE OF WATER

I remember driving down Dort Highway. It seemed that the lights were extremely bright and blaring in my eyes. Each light I reached turned red, and this was the one time I did not want to be late.

"Come on! Come on! People, I am in a fricken' hurry!" I screamed while my glove covered hands griped the steering wheel of my cherry red Pontiac G6. "I just can't be late for this thing!"

I didn't know what to expect when I got to the bariatric center. What would everyone look like? Would they greet me at the door? Will the doctor give enough information? There were so many questions swimming through my brain that it was hard to concentrate, and I missed my turn into the institute.

"Damn!"

After making some adjustments and many left turns, I pulled into the parking lot of the bariatric center, and the gloves on my hands were already drenched with sweat. Most would wonder why so much stress because to the common person this was just a seminar, an informational gathering. No, not for me. This was my first true step, and tonight would help me make the biggest decision I have ever made in my life. This was a step toward my health, and I wasn't completely sure I was ready for this adventure.

After entering the sliding door and peering around the corner, a kindly looking middle aged woman in light pink medical scrubs almost bumped into me while walking to the informational table.

"Don't be scared, sweetie. Come on over so we can take care of you."

There was already a gathering around the table of people of every background, young and old. I patiently waited my turn behind three other people, a strawberry blonde, a older gentleman in a pea coat, and an elderly woman with a cane, who were gathering handouts and placing them in their folders. After what seemed to be an eternity, I was at the head of the line.

"Hello and welcome! Could we have your name so we can check your registration?"

I nervously mumbled my name and a younger blond scanned her French tip painted finger down a list lying on the table in front of her.

"Well, hello Jessyca! What a unique spelling of your name!"

I did the standard reply that I have used millions of times before, "Mom wanted to be creative." My mother gave me the unique spelling of my first name because she saw it in a book. She said she knew it would fit me, even before I was born. Mom always liked to remind me that I was different in so many ways, from my speech to my outlooks on life. She was right, and I love it when people comment on the uniqueness of my name.

Next I received a black folder, filled with information, handouts on the procedure and the many smiles from the staff that were there for support. The last item I received was my lifesaver, a free bottle of water.

Now, many would say, "What is the big deal of a free bottle of water?"

Honestly, my throat and mouth were as dry as the Sahara. My teeth were chattering, and I began to do my nervous tick of grinding my teeth as soon as I walked through the sliding door. The bottled water was my revival source, by nourishment, and most importantly, my distracter. As long as I continued to sip on that bottle of water, I wouldn't have to speak to anyone and share my story. Thank God for that bottle of water.

The room was arranged with simple division in the middle, with seven rows and six seats in each row. I sat in the second to last row near the edge so that I could have a clear view for the presentation. There was a screen placed in the front of the room, and many of the seats were already filled. I looked at the other eager faces in the room and realized I was actually one of the smallest people there, which I must say, was incredibly odd, but not comforting. How could I be proud of being the smallest of the big people? While examining the other people there, I noticed a critic on the other side of the room. An older woman, wearing polyester grey pants was staring me down. She actually shot me a dirty look, and then shifted over to her husband, who was leaning on his wooden cane. After she finished sharing her secret, he turned, looked at me and said, "Hump". I felt bewildered due to not knowing what was said, but I did know she was not pleased with something dealing with me. I leaned down, dug through my purse, and took out my favorite purple pen to take notes.

The introduction for the seminar was quite simple. One nurse stood in front of us and gave us a hearty greeting. She was small in figure and wearing cartoon medical scrubs. She had bouncy, blonde hair and designer looking glasses, and she made me feel comfortable.

She pleasantly went through the agenda, and did small jokes between the documentation that would make the seminar run smoothly. She then said "welcome" again and leaned over for the lecture presenter placed next to the overhead. She announced that the doctor would speak to us for a short time.

As the doctor stepped forward, everyone adjusted in their seat to pay attention to the expert in this field. Dr. F. was an olive skinned fellow dawned in a white doctor lab coat. He wasn't smiling when he stepped forward, and seemed so tall that his head could touch the ceiling. His presence frightened me slightly, especially knowing that he might be the man to make miracles happen with my health.

Dr. F. took the lecture presenter and greeted us dryly to begin his speech. He then said that he would go through and discuss each procedure, and extended his hand to click the lecture presenter.

The slide didn't move.

He clicked again.

Nothing.

The presenter had failed to work.

Dr. F. fidgeted with the remote and pressed the button multiple times, but again, the slide would not change. He tilted his head, held the lecture presenter close to his face and then said, "Well, I guess one of my nurses has broken the presenter."

I snickered lightly at that comment, and dipped my chin to my chest so those around me wouldn' hear my giggle. Dr. F. turned and faced the crowd, "I guess there will be no presentation today since my staff had decided to break the presenter. Shame on all of you nurses, breaking all these people's hearts!"

More giggles came, and so did a more comfortable atmosphere. Dr. F. was actually quite a cheerful man, who was quick witted in a time of crisis, and I liked that. He did his presentation smoothly, even with the technology issues, explained the differences in surgeries, passed around a model of the two types of gastric banding, and finished with multiple jokes and comforting words.

The cheery blond nurse stepped forward once again when Dr. F. had completed the information. She cheered for everyone because we came out on an icy December night. She concluded by saying if we wanted to schedule time for the doctor to stop by the table and set an appointment.

I knew this was the right decision. I walked up to the table and set my examination date with the doctor. Things were falling into place.

And now to share the news.

SHARING THE NEWS

I was unsure how people would take the news about my decision to have bariatric surgery. As I stated before, I didn't care about most people's opinion, but I had to be realistic, people were going to have something to say. Some people will be happy, some people will frown on the idea, and some people would think I was just plain crazy. I was most worried about telling my parents, who mean the world to me, about the surgery. I knew that I needed to have an opening up session with someone I trusted before talking to my parents, and I had that with my best friend on earth, my partner in crime, Bill.

Before I get into my first opening up session about becoming a gastric band member, you need to know some background information about my relationship with Mr. Opinion, better known as Bill. He is the one person in this world that could tell me to shut up and I would have nothing to say back. He is the best friend that everyone needs, the one who will hold you when you are crying and tell you it is going to be alright. He is the one who will whip you into shape if you are not living up to your potential. He is the one who has you try crazy things, and then make fun of you for going along with his decision of insanity. He will listen carefully, and be brutally honest when he needs to be. I love him more than words can express because he is the total package in human existence.

I met Bill at a football meeting. In my past life, I was a football team owner (which is a book in itself, but essential in explaining the tale of the meeting of Bill and I). Bill was hired by my father and uncle to work on the broadcasting team for our football squad. I knew very little about him, except that he did a great interview and wore a suit when meeting with my father and uncle, which intrigued me because one of my serious weaknesses in life (other than brownies) is an attractive man in a suit. He was the only one who went the extra mile in his interview according to the boys, and I wanted to get a look at him and see what he was all about. When he walked into the meeting he did not disappoint my expectations. Once again he was nicely dressed, tan, and one fine-looking Caucasian man to stare at.

During the meeting I couldn't figure out if Bill was super confident or arrogant, and it irritated me to no end. He sat there with this superior demeanor, like he knew he was the man at what he did, which I didn't know if I should respect or turn my nose up to. But a powerful and confident man is hard to turn away from, and Bill was indeed that.

We caught each other's glance a couple times in the meeting, and when it was my turn to run the show and explain the expectations and the drive for everyone to reach perfection, he stared me down…hard. We later found out we were both puzzled and studying one another, because we both knew there was something different about each other. Bill was intrigued at the fact that there was a female owner who knew more about football than the average man. To top it off, he thought I was an attractive black chick, which, as it turned out, was his biggest weakness. As time went by, Bill and I became close, much closer than anyone could imagine since he ended up moving to Flint and spending many crazy years under the same roof as me.

We have lived together for multiple years, but aren't together, which I totally understand outsiders raising an eyebrow at the notion. Even odder, I can say that he is the one man I truly love outside of my family, but I am not IN love with him. We often are mistaken as a married couple, and we both shake our heads at the notion. Our relationship is quite complicated and odd, but it works for us, and it makes our friendship stronger than most. I rely on him to be honest, loyal, and caring when I need him to be, and he hasn't let me down. Bill, at the point of the gastric band opening up session, had already taken care of me after one surgery when I had a tumor, and if I did the band, he would be my sole caregiver during a major transition in my life, which is a lot to ask. We had to talk about my decision, and I had to speak to Bill before anyone else. He is a key component of my success and my life.

So one Saturday morning before attending the bariatric center seminar, I decided to share the news with Bill and hear his comments and concerns. We were relaxing in my bedroom, both sprawled out on my queen size bed and watching TV, which is a regular accordance on lazy weekends.

"Bill, I've been thinking about something really serious lately, and need you to listen," I stated.

"If you're thinking about something nasty, I don't want to hear it."

I also need to state that Bill is one of the biggest smart asses you will ever meet (which proves I was right on the "arrogant" analysis at the football meeting) and occasionally I want to ring his neck for his quick wit, but his quick thinking was also something I adored about him. I replied as I usually did, I kicked him on his side.

"I'm serious, I need you to listen. I am thinking about making a life changing decision, a very serious decision."

Bill's 6'3" frame sat up, turned, faced me, and he officially put on his serious face, which consisted on him squinting his hazel eyes for a moment, a rub of his salt and pepper beard, followed by tucking his hands on his lap, and slightly leaning forward.

I began to tell Bill of my Internet search and my voice quivered when I came to my final statement,

"I think I am going to do this banding thing. I need to do it."

He frowned and he looked inquisitively at me.

"Are you doing this for looks or for your health?"

I thought this was a valid question. I didn't know how it was to be thin girl. I never have been "skinny", but that wasn't my motivation, although it would be a nice benefit.

"Bill, I have had high blood pressure for over a decade. I have cheated death and survived a blood clot. I have heard time and time again to just lose some weight and everything will be fine. Well, I can't lose the weight, not with diet plans, not with exercise, not with cutting out fast food completely. I need help, permanent help. If I keep waiting, my body will continue to slowly die. What do you think?"

Bill leaned back and rested his body on the bed frame. His eyes were piercing through me, and I began to feel nervous for his reply. I knew he had wisdom for me because he did his traditional actions when it came to trivial matters; he closed his eyes, took a deep breath, and then tilted his head before he spoke.

"Jes, I think it's a good idea. I think it's the right thing to do. If anyone deserves years of being healthy, it's you. You deserve this and I'm there for you."

I took a deep breath and felt a sense of relief; someone was in my corner on this adventure. Even if everyone else thought I was crazy, I had my friend to go through this ordeal with me. As I was enjoying the moment, I heard Bill speaking to me again.

"If you are going to do this, I want you to tell how this thing works. I wanna understand how everything works, even if it grosses me out. And I can only hope you don't become an annoying, skinny bitch."

That was a typical reply from my best friend. Bill offered to go with me, but I refused, I wanted to make this decision on my own. Plus, I didn't want him to start joking around with me and I start giggling at such a serious event.

After basically sliding home from the meeting due to yet another Flint, MI, ice storm, I walked in my house, hung up my coat, and heard Bill call for me to come have a talk. I took my informational folder into his room and this time, settled on the end of his bed. I curled his black comforter around my legs and took a deep, cleansing breath. I told him everything, my feelings, the information, my impressions of the staff and doctor. I finished after sharing with him that I had set my doctor's appointment date to start the process.

"So, is this really what you want? Because there is no going back once you start this."

I knew that question was coming, and I went over and over my decision while driving home.

I nodded my head with a small grin. "I am ready for this. It's what I want. I am going do it."

"Well heffa, I am right there with you."

Once again, there was a kick to his side.

THE FAMILY

The next group to discuss the surgery with was my parents. Their opinion was very important to me. Their opinion would not change my mind this time, but it is still important to hear their point of view. I know that they would think about things at a different level.

My mother is the one that everyone leans on. When something is wrong within the family, she is the one to call. She is the icon of understanding, the caregiver that everyone wants and needs. I must also add that she is very light complexion, beyond pretty to everyone, and has the label of being a "diva". She will not be around people unless she has on her make-up, her outfit, and, most importantly, her hair. She is the queen of cuteness to young and old, male and female, and has always been my plus size idol. She also has struggled with weight issues, and has worked to make herself healthier. Her weight came from medications. Despite being plus size, she was close to four inches taller than I, and always carried her weight well.

My father is better known as "Coach" Mathews, and telling him about this choice would be a completely different ordeal than telling my mother. He is average height, with a glare that could kill anyone when a bad football play was made. Many of my major problems with my weight come from my father's bloodline, because there is "uniqueness" on being built like a Mathews. I am built exactly like my father. He is a man with the widest shoulders that you have ever seen; they are shoulders that you would imagine Atlas to have, since that mythological icon carried the sins of the world upon those heavy shoulders. Everything on him was strong and large:

his arms, calves, even his neck. He is built like a football coach, and has a physical presence that demanded respect. This is all well and good when you are a man, but when you are a 5'4" female, these physical characteristics can work against you.

As I stated before, the real obstacle would be my father. The main reason is I am daddy's little girl, and he wants to protect me from anything, and everything, that could harm me. Being a coach means that you plan everything to be perfect. You're precise and many times, obsessive. I know, since I am a coach myself. There is no room for error when you have a coach's mind, and surgery has the strong possibility of error. My father would think about the surgeon "fumbling" the surgery on me, or calling the wrong play, or losing the big game. He wouldn't be willing to lose me because of the mistake by some doctor.

My parents had been away visiting my sister in Alabama when I had gone to the bariatric center's seminar, which made things easier that I could go and make up my own mind. When they returned, I went over with my information before visiting their house. I pulled into the drive way and sat for a couple minutes before walking up to the porch, and gently knocking on the front door on the medium house in one of the quietest parts of Flint.

The discussion went pretty well, despite the look of distain on my father's face. My mother, was overjoyed with the news, and was my biggest cheerleader in the beginning stages of making this decision. She sat intently, nodding her head when I explained my reasoning for doing the surgery at this point in my life. She interrupted (as she often did with any topic) at times with valid questions, and insisted on keeping the folder of information that the hospital gave me so that she could read over the facts of the surgery a couple times for complete understanding.

My mother is a medical information junkie, the one who watches surgeries and odd documentaries on TV. There were many times that she would call me late in the evening to watch some oddity show on her favorite channels. She liked stories about unique births and people coping with mental disorders and making it in our stressful society. I think she mostly did this because she suffered from bipolar disorder, and felt the more information she stored, the more she could cope. So, it didn't surprise me that she wanted to cipher through all the information about this surgery.

My father, on the other hand, was quite quiet. He sat staring into space on the white, plush couch placed in the front room, directly in front of his fire place. I could tell that he disapproved of my decision, but he knew I wouldn't change my mind with my blabbering. Like many of the characteristics I had obtained from his family line, he was stubborn, a common thread in the Mathews's family line. The only thing I can remember him saying in the conversations was, "If this is what you want to do, go ahead." It wasn't in an approving tone.

It was a month later when my father and I had a real conversation about this surgery idea. He came over to my home to pick up my laptop to do some work for his online broadcasting company. When he arrived at my house he was wearing his usual coaching gear, a long t-shirt, hat, and warm up pants. He simply came into the house, settled into the computer chair and started the conversation.

"So, I have been thinking about this whole surgery thing with you. It makes me nervous, but I understand why you want to do it. You are stopping the chances of disease that runs ramped in our family. Truthfully, I don't blame you."

My father had in that month's time found out that he was diabetic, and was having serious struggles with his sugar level. He had begun injection after injection just weeks after I told them for the first time that I wanted to have the Lapband done. There were many trips to the doctor, and being forced to change his lifestyle, which was a struggle. When I think about the timing of these events I always made me wonder if God did this on purpose. To have such a negative of my father's health turning for the worse and me wanting to make my health go toward the positive could not be a coincidence.

In any event, getting his approval made me feel much better about the situation. He had shared the news with my grandparents, Burnie and Evon, who, surprisingly, thought it was the best idea I had ever had. My mother told my grandma, Edna, and her side of the family, and they agreed.

The only other people that I went into an in-depth conversation about having the surgery were my quiet brother, Chris, and my sister, nurse-to-be, Angi. My brother made it clear from listening to me speak to my parents that I should just do what makes me happy. That's his style. He will speak up if he thinks you're being an idiot, but does not rock the boat if he sees you have made your decision. The conversation with Angi was a tad different.

Angi had decided to go to school for nursing, and had become a medical junkie like mom. She would be the one to read every medical journal and website and give her strong opinion. She was constantly studying and juggling my three nephews, but she always had time to give her opinion on anything, even if you didn't want to hear it. After a long discussion, and hearing her opinion, she gave her approval and said it was a great idea. It was time to move forward.

JUMPING THROUGH HOOPS

One thing that they do not share with you when you decide to take this journey is you will jump through multiple hoops. I must put the disclaimer that everyone has their own "hoops" to jump through. One should call their insurance company to find out what circus quest they want you to go through. I was lucky, my insurance wasn't that difficult in the matter, and the majority of my surgery was covered by my insurance company. I didn't really have to worry about the money issue of surgery, but know that most people do, and it can be quite costly. My insurance company insisted on a doctor recommendation, a surgeon recommendation, and, the last major "hoop", a psychiatric exam.

My first doctor's meeting was with the same man from the center, Dr. F. It was quite brief, and he was more direct with our one-on-one meeting. He looked over my major health issues, my current weight, and the medications I was taking. He agreed that I was the right candidate for gastric banding. He explained how the process worked and why I was a good candidate. It was the first time that I had to accept the words "morbidly obese." I was morbidly obese, no matter what anyone said or the cute words people could use. I was in danger of dying at a young age, in danger for more diseases and disorders, and this could be a way to save my life.

Hearing that information from the terrified me, but I knew I needed to hear it. I had thought about those words coming out his mouth, but it was different to hear it said to me directly in the face. It helped me put a confirmation on this whole idea.

The doctor continued to tell me about some of the positives of me having the surgery at my age. My skin should bounce back better, which means me not having to have too much skin hanging from my body, or the need to have skin surgically removed. I would be able to be more active, and although the weight would drop less than having the bigger bariatic surgeries, but in the upcoming years, I would be way smaller and way healthier. I told him that everything sounded right, and I ask only a couple questions before I heard my last set of directions.

As I stated before, my family doctor was not a fan of bariatric surgery. I have gone to the same doctor my entire life. My doctor always listens, but he will state his opinion when need be. He is a thin man, with small glasses that tend to slide down to the end of his nose. I loved talking my medical man, Doctor Dolven. He has gone through so many different issues with my family, especially my parents and I.

I was extremely nervous to talk with him about it again, but there was a key member of his staff that helped me have the guts to discuss it. She was a kindly nurse, with short hair and glasses, and she had a grandmother appeal to me. She was always in the office when I came in and always very positive, no matter how sick anyone was. She came into the room after I was called back, and asked why I was in the see the doctor. I told her that I was considering having gastric banding surgery, and she paused her writing in my chart and looked up. She too knew that my doctor was not a fan of having that surgery, and she stated her opinion to me.

"You stand your ground, girl. You tell him what you think and why you think it, and you don't change your mind. I have a daughter that had surgery for your issue, and she is a new person. She doesn't regret it, and I supported her from day one. You tell him that you are ready to be healthy, and that you know what's best for you."

She was the one to give me the strength to look the doctor in the eye and say "I am going to do this procedure." I didn't ask permission, I told him why I was having it and said that this was going to happen. My doctor looked at me stunned and smiled after I was finished. He stated that he understood, and did the paperwork for the surgery. He stressed to do what the surgeon says because there are many people who don't follow orders, and to make sure to tell him everything that was going on. I made it through the easiest medical hoop, but the harder hoop, a visit to a psychiatrist, was to come next.

I had never been to a shrink, and the thought of going to one made me very nervous. I couldn't have the surgery without his/her approval, which meant one person could make or break my dreams of a new life. I didn't want to be analyzed; I didn't want to share my inner most fat secrets. Some were so painful, and so deep that the last thing I wanted to do was spit my fat soul open again. But there was no way around it, I had to be examined and it had to be determined that I was mentally fit enough for this surgery to happen.

My appointment was set in May. The idea of seeing a shrink worked me up so that I took the day off of work for my appointment. I knew there was no way I could concentrate on teaching high schoolers with the upcoming event of Jessyca being dissected by some strange man sitting behind a desk.

I had a vision of me being forced to lie on a couch and talk until I cried about my fat flashbacks, and it made me sick. What would he ask? Would I say something wrong? What if I didn't pass the exam?

The first bad sign was I couldn't find his office. I found the building easily, but there were several offices in the building and I had no idea where to go. The first office was another shrink, and they told me to head to the other end of the building. They failed to tell me where the door to the far wing was, and I passed it three times before I actually found it. I didn't even find the stupid door until someone in the dentist office came out and assisted me. So I was almost late (which I can't stand being) when I walked through Dr. W.'s door.

The secretary was pleasant, but it didn't help my uneasiness. I was handed a clip board with papers to fill out, and she told me to turn in the profile documents that they sent me in the mail. The most disturbing part of this process was the profile they sent me in the mail. The questions started off with the typical information: name, address, phone, age. I had written this information tons of times during banding process, but then the questions changed.

I was asked when I lost my virginity, if I had a homosexual experience, experimented with drugs, how often I drank, if I had been abused, and other incredibly personal items. I was stunned at what they wanted to know. What does my age of loss virginity have to do with weight loss surgery? I was outraged, and I called my mother about it.

"I guess they just wanna make sure nothing in your closet will get in the way of your success," was her reply.

After finishing the papers on the clipboard I handed it, along with all my embarrassing answers on the profile, to the secretary.

"The doctor will be with you in a couple minutes Jessyca. Just sit and relax."

Relax. How can I relax knowing this man is going to look at me under a microscope? I was shaking with nervous energy, and after what seemed to be an eternity, my name was called to the back.

Dr. W. looked like the typical middle aged, Caucasian American. His hairline was creeping backwards, and he was sporting a sweater that you would imagine Bill Cosby would wear on television. He shook my hand firmly, and then settled into his plush, tan doctor chair. His office was not anything flashy; actually it was rather plain, with awards and small knick knacks on the shelves and on his desk. He stared directly at me with a cheerful tone and he spoke and asked some basic questions to get to know me. After a short visit, the doctor explained that I would be moved to another room for the examination. I started to feel uneasy, and had visions of me being in room with one single light shining down on me, and being quizzed on my most intimate details to get a stamp of "yes" or "no" to surgery. Instead of being lead into a interrogation room, I was placed in a small room not much larger than a closest, which contained just a chair, desk, and a computer.

I was asked to take a personality test on the computer with over 150 questions. I simply had to rate the statement on a scale, 1-5, from strongly agree (5) to strongly disagree (1). I wasn't allowed to skip any of the statements, and I was supposed to answer each one honestly, and without over thinking the question. Dr. W. finished up with the last set of directions on the test and asked if I understood. After I comprehended the task at hand, I settled into the chair and the door was closed.

Now, some of the statements were really stupid. One asked, "I love to play with puzzles". What the hell does this have to do with my mental state for this surgery? I rolled my eyes and clicked to move to the next question. As the test continued, the statements became harder, and more complicated to answer, then came the questions that made me think about myself.

"Have you ever wanted to just get away?"

"Do you like to have everything in order?"

"Have you ever thought about suicide?"

"I tend to eat when I am depressed."

They were questions and statements I didn't want to click that I strongly agreed with, but to click anything else would be lying, which I am terrible at. My hands began to sweat, I began to grit my teeth, and I knew I was not dealing with the pressure of the test well. I stopped taking the test for a moment.

I sat there and examined myself. Should I be honest in answering this test, or should I put what I think they want to hear? I stared at the wall instead of the bright screen on the computer. What would count for what they wanted to hear? I realized I was over complicating the matter, and the process was making my head hurt. Finally, I made up my mind. I needed to be honest, and deal with the consequences of the test. If this man comes to me and says I am too crazy to have this surgery it would crush me, but at least I would have a clear conscience. I wiped my hands on my pants, took a deep breath, and continued clicking away at the questions probing into my soul.

My fear of failing the test came from the history of mental illness in my family. There have been issues with depression, bi-polar disorder, among other things, but I had never been diagnosed with any disorder. I had an extreme fear of suddenly been labeled, of being the next in line with the family to have mental disorders that required patience and medication. I couldn't hide from a disorder if it came out from taking this test, and I didn't want to deal with those issues if it did show that I had a problem.

I took another deep breath and continued to click away at the statements. Finally, I came to the end, and I was instructed to go back into the waiting room until I was called back again to speak to the doctor. I had to stay in the waiting room until my results were calculated and it was driving me crazy. I thought about my answers, I thought about this opportunity, and I thought about the possibility that I would be told that this was not for me. In the midst of my daydreaming I heard my name called to come back and speak with the doctor.

He motioned for me to sit down and looked over my papers while I sat there nervously fidgeting in my chair. Finally, the doctor placed the papers on his desk, cleared his throat, and then looked me directly in the face.

"So, Jessyca. How long have you been OCD?"

I almost said "What the Hell!" out loud to the man. Instead I said, "Pardon me?"

"Oh Jessyca, you, my dear, you suffer from Obsessive Compulsive Disorder."

He explained the disorder to me and asked me questions to help me see that I had this issue. He asked if I am obsessed with being on time, with perfection, with things being my way, with organization of everything at home or at work, the feeling of failure if things were not perfect. I was nodding with each statement, of course I focused on these things, but that was not OCD according to what I had seen. I have taught OCD kids who struggle with behavior, and watched reality television shows of people who had to lock the door five times each time they stood at their door. That was not me.

He began to explain the branch of OCD that I had. I just thought that showed I had a strong personality, but I guess to others it would seem a tad obsessive. I couldn't argue this logic. This view was new to me, and all the things he said were describing me.

He next asked if I had gone through manic phrases in my life. This, I honestly could not attest to. I had times where I was filled with energy and was overly active, but I didn't know if that defined me being manic. I had seen my mother in her manic phases, and they were not pretty to look at. I remember her sometimes cooking at three in the morning, or waking up to staying up all night cleaning. I had never done that, and I honestly couldn't answer his question. After the examination I called Bill to ask if I had a manic episode since we lived together. He fell silent, then giggled, and replied, "You indeed have." I found out that my cleaning at times had been quite manic to my friend, and I had no idea. I just thought I was being tidy.

After being analyzed to death a fear hit me. Am I crazy? Am I unfit to have this surgery? He hadn't said "yes" or "no" yet. Finally, I received my news.

"Jessyca, there is no reason for you to not be mentally stable for surgery. Despite your small OCD issues, you are a mentally healthy person, but I do want you to keep this business card in case you need to speak to someone after surgery. It can, and will be mentally draining, and sometimes you will need to speak to someone."

He handed me a card of a psychiatrist that had actually gone through the same surgery I did, and said if I ever felt that mentally needed help to call her. I place the card in my wallet, and it is still there in case I need her.

The paperwork would only take a couple days, and then they would call me with my surgery date. I had made it through a giant "hoop" and now the hard part of my journey had begun.

FAT FLASHBACK-RED LIGHT SPECIAL WITH RKB

I have always been able to fake that that I am a harmonious woman of confidence, toughness, and immovability. People would assume that I was incapable of being broken in times of trouble and that my feet were always planted firmly in the ground. I spoke with my head held high, and I walked with a swagger of conceit and confidence most days, which, I can admit now, was a complete lie before surgery. I believed this behavior would keep people at bay, and that no one would really question me if I were feeling alright or truly happy. Being the girl with the cold glare and firm stance always seemed to work on people, and no one questioned it. That is, no one questioned it until I met RKB.

There has never been a person in my life to see me the way Randy (known as RKB to me) has. It has always puzzled me that he was the one to see the "true" me, and had the ability to tell me the right things at the right time. RKB didn't just see me. He saw THROUGH me. He saw through the bull shit that I played daily with others, and that man is still able to pick me apart today. It took me some time to see that he completely understood my feelings on everything and my relevance on earth.

RKB and I met many years ago over my soccer parents, The Dresser's, household. We were both hired to coach girls in a soccer program. Oddly enough, we both grew up in the same district, and had family members cross paths for multiple years. Yet, we had never met until a cold, snow-filled February evening. RKB was close to 6'2", far from having swarthy skin with his incredible light complexion, and was the supreme specimen of a physically fit man. I almost didn't want to look at him for a second time when he first entered the Dresser's home. I had fear that the swirling dirty thoughts running through my mind and my glaze would be completely inappropriate. I can say now with a devilish grin that the first thoughts to cross my mind were, "There is no way a man of this level of sexy would EVER talk to me, even if we are coaching for the same team!"

RKB strolled directly over to me and reached for my hand in a pleasant greeting. I fumbled off the snug cushions of the Dresser's couch to stand and shake his hand properly. I had to be professional, despite wanting to act like a school girl and gaze at the attractive man I would be spending spring soccer seasons with on a regular basis.

Our hands met.

I flinched at the frigid temperature of his palm, and shrunk away. He smirked slightly, and stated with a rhapsody of words that were as cool as the air that rushed in during this cold winter evening, "You must excuse me, but remember, cold hands, warm heart."

After letting go of teenage girl behavior and getting to actually know the man, I have found that RKB is the warmest hearted man I have ever met. He ended up being there as my friend during some of the worst times of battling with my weight. I was at my heaviest when we coached together, and he never made me feel less than pretty.

We spent many hours giggling on the phone or being cobbled together on bus rides to different soccer games. With seeing each other every day, I found myself sharing my pain with him. He gave me one of the best gifts that you can receive in life. He didn't just hear me, he listened to me. And he answered with words of inspiration, care, and and hope. RKB was unique. He was one of three men (of course am including Bill and Damiekco in this grouping) in my life that I felt never had a problem with my weight. His compliments, encouragement, his listening ear and gusto helped me during my darkest times.

Simply put, I adore him.

There were multiple defining moments with RKB and me.

During the high times of my friendship with Randy, I had a serious back problem. The pain sometimes would be crippling, causing me to shuffle around my house gritting my teeth and creasing my brow in anguish. I would also feel this way some days after coaching.

I remember one road trip from Owosso. After the game I was in such bad shape that the pain jetted from my lower back, down my legs, and even shocked each one of my toes. I was in such pain that in my search for relief, I lay across the front seat of the bus, across from RKB and Coach Dresser. I thought that if I stretched out, I could have some relief because I didn't have any of my medication with me.

I lay there, feeling like an oddball with my face resting sideways on the musty bus seat. My eyes were closed tightly the majority of the time, but for a brief moment I did open them and sat half way up to examine my surroundings. He was looking intensely over at me. I laid back, wondering why he was studying me so closely. The bus rambled down many back roads, and the pain became more intense. I felt an ache percolate down my tailbone. I bit down hard on my back teeth to resist crying out from the discomfort.

For a brief moment, the pain subsided, and I felt something. There was a hand resting on the crook of my knee. I felt the hand then travel downward and then there was a soft stroke on my leg. I heard him whisper, "You alright, JMeezy?" which was the pet name he gave me during the season. Oddly enough, he still uses it 'til this day.

I didn't answer him.

RKB has always had the ability to know when my health was in turmoil. I really don't understand how he is been able to know this because pain was part of my daily life during the times I coached with him, but no one else on that bus had a clue. RKB knew I was physically suffering, even when I was too stubborn to admit that there was a problem.

After arriving back to the high school, I struggled down the bus steps and tried to do a limp-like toddle to my car. Randy ran to catch me. He later shared that his plan was for me not to even drive home due to me looking like I could barely walk. I wanted to get to my car as quick as I could because I felt the tears starting to form in my eyes as the pain increased.

I couldn't cry in front of him.

I had shown weakness to him in sharing stories, but I couldn't bare the idea of being weak enough to cry in front of him. Randy caught my arm, stopping me from opening the car door, and with anxious eyes stared at me.

"JMezzy, I'm worried about you. Don't lie to me about being alright. Do you need me?"

This was the one time I did lie to RKB. I said that I was "fine", but I was in immense pain. The fact that I made it home was a miracle. I remember the frustration that raged inside me that evening because I was convinced the back issues were from the weight. It frustrated me. I found out later that I was right. The weight was making a serious problem with my back. I still have some problems, but losing the access weight made it easier for me to deal with.

I don't know how I did it, but I struggled to work the next day. No student noticed my limp when I did my lesson, and I wasn't questioned by any co-workers. I made it through the day without one person noticing I wasn't 100 percent. During my 6th hour, I checked my cell and he had called. Minutes after the school bell rung, I picked up my phone and he had called again. I dialed his number.

There was a hostile tone when he answered. I questioned what the issue was, and he forcefully told me the tale of his day and worrying about me. He had called my cell three times…and emailed…and called the house phone and spoke to my father because he was looking for me. I found it comical. He spoke to me through a clenched jaw, and I knew that he was not amused.

"How can a woman, who was crippled the night before, drag into work the next day?" he questioned.

"The team needs to practice. If I stay home, we can't get the team ready for the next game," I replied.

He snickered. "JMezzy, you are indeed super human."

His follow up statement made a grin appear to my face. He simply said, "I'm proud of you."

I appreciated the comment, and felt at that moment that RKB was a lifetime friend, and would always watch out for me because he was my set of watchful eyes with my health.

The best times between the two of us were always spent in a special place, my car. In my red Saturn was the place where we would have deep discussions about soccer, share dirty secrets, and talked about what we both wanted in our lives. I never felt that I couldn't share anything I thought with RKB, and he was always completely honest with me.

I believed him when he said I was pretty, that I was special, and that I would make someone a wonderful wife someday. He just-- understood. The fact that he could do this would terrify me. Many times I would get so nervous that I would cower back in my driver's side seat and tap my manicured hands rapidly on the gear shift when we were sitting in the driveway of his home. Even though we were just friends, he found a way to make me blush in these discussions. But I needed someone to remind me that despite my weight, I was a beautiful person inside and out.

One warm May afternoon, I was having one of my nervous moments at a red light near a busy intersection. I was tapping profusely on the gear shift, staring straight ahead into the sunset so that I wouldn't have to show my shyness because RKB was giving me yet another one of his "You are wonderful" pep talks.

Suddenly, RKB reached over and gently took my hand. Once again, just the same as the day we first met; an icy-cold rush went through my veins from his palm. I remember turning my head slightly toward him while he clasped his fingers inside of mine. This was different than the first time in the fact that I wasn't filled with dirty thoughts and uncomfortable introductions. Holding his hand the second time was much more precious. Music was playing softly on the radio and the sun was a beautiful shade that could only be appreciated when it leaves for the evening to rest. The moment seemed so perfect.

"Jes, you don't have to be nervous about being special. A man should be able to spend a lifetime saying how wonderful and beautiful you are. If he wants to, you let him."

I was afraid for him to let my hand go. It was one of the times in my life that I didn't feel fat and I didn't downgrade that I was around someone who thought I was worth paying attention to. I was beautiful and most important, I was happy. My friend RKB always made me happy.

That is, until…

STARVATION

One of the hardest things that I had to go through before having the surgery was the liquid fast. I have been told that each medical institution handles this differently, so I can only speak to the steps asked of me from My hospital. Hardship number one is purchasing the protein food package that Hurley requires you to have. I could not just go to the store and buy the protein shakes on the shelves, I had to order a package over the Internet that had all the required items to ensure a successful surgery.

The package cost almost $300! I almost passed out when I saw the cost on my Internet order. All that money for a liquid diet? I hadn't had an expensive dinner in years because I couldn't afford that high class treatment, and now I was about to spend hundreds of dollars on powdered substances that would be added to milk! And to make matters worse, I had to add soy milk to my mixtures due to being lactose intolerant (I have never been able to drink milk. It is a youthful experience that I cannot share with others, if I tried to drink a glass of milk, I would be sick as a dog), and that meant spending even more money on the high class measures to prevent me spending many of hours on the porcelain high chair known as my toilet in my pretty bathroom. Soy milk is not cheap people, and neither of weight loss.

Luckily, I decided to have the surgery as soon as school ended, and I had received a coaching check for my spring season, so I was able to order the pre-surgery diet kit without any major issues.

The diet consisted of my choice of three flavor shakes and one flavor of gelatin. I, being a traditionalist, chose the classic flavors:

vanilla, chocolate and strawberry. My choice for gelatin was cherry because I figured there was no way that cherry could taste awful. The package arrived three days before I had to begin doing my fast in a big white box, with a cheerful message of congratulations on making a decision to improve my life. There was a free gift of a mixing cup for my shakes, which I thought was precious at the beginning stages of getting ready for the fast.

My final days before the fast were filled with me eating anything I could. I felt that I needed to do a farewell tour to all the foods that I adored before taking on this challenge. By this time, I had shared the news with the co-workers that I had lunch with. I figured that word would travel about my choice by telling the lunch room crew about getting the "GB" because there is no such thing as a secret at CAHS. One day I had Chinese, the next day I had a gyro with fries (with extra onion). Then there was the day with the sub with everything I could think of on it, with a side of nacho cheese chips. I called it "Jes's Final Food Tour", and enjoyed sugar filled treats throughout the final tour.

The last day of official food was pizza. Oh, how I love pizza. I remember having that last meal, and getting nervous about starting the liquid fast. But the nervousness turned to excitement, and I was positive about starting the liquid diet to lose some weight before starting my surgery. This was the last happy day I had for about two weeks.

I think that the best phrase to explain the liquid diet is simple, "It totally sucked ass." It was one of the hardest things I had to do, and it made me into a bitter, hostile, monster. I think that after you hear about the ordeal, you will understand why.

During the liquid fast, you are required to drink five shakes a day and to have the "treat" of one gelatin dessert. The shakes don't taste bad; actually they were pretty good for the first couple of days. The vanilla was my favorite because it tasted like cake batter, with chocolate, which tasted like a candy bar, was a very close second. The cherry dessert was the most disgusting gelatin I had ever experienced! It was gritty, and had an after taste that stayed on your tongue for hours. I hated it so much, but I had eat it, so I literally chanted, "Think happy thoughts" while I choking it down.

Taste wasn't the major suckiness of doing the liquid fast. It was the lack of chewing. It's strange, but humans have an obsession with chewing things. We love chewing our food, and having those miscellaneous things like gum to satisfy our oral fixations. If you do meal after meal without chewing, your mind feels that something is wrong. My need to chew started on day two, and my mind started to wander toward the forbidden thoughts of the pleasures of the foods I ate before the fast. I realized that doing the food tour was probably one of the most damaging things I could have done for my psychological state. It made my food cravings during the fast more intense, and it was a serious battle not to fall into the world of food temptation.

I was also asked to drink 64 ounces of water a day, which made me pee so much that I didn't even want to leave the bathroom during the day. So, all I did for 14 days was drink. I always had a cup in my hand, and I sipped throughout the entire day, and it irritated me to no end.

I did well for about three days according to Bill, and then I went to "hungry bitch" mode (his words, not mine), where everything and everyone annoyed me, especially drinking the shakes. He jokes about my worst day, Day Five, when I started counting the number of food commercials during a quiz show. They did seven commercials in a row of delicious burgers, chicken, and subs, and there I was, sipping on a chocolate protein shake, with my snack being a damn sugar-free frozen treat. My reply to noticing the stockpile of food commercials was simple.

"Do they have to have all these fucking food commercials in a row? It's fucking brutal!!!"

His body jumped from my outburst, but he didn't reply. He later shared with me that he didn't want to be attacked. This was the moment that I changed. I was livid all the time, and turned into a hungry, crabby monster during the shake fast according to Bill. I know he wasn't making it up, I was miserable chugging down those five shakes a day. I actually had food withdrawal and developed hunger headaches, and I complained the whole time to my best friend, and, with a smile (most of the time), Bill listened and was supportive.

Bill tried to sneak and eat late at night so that I wouldn't have to watch him eat during this time, but it didn't work. God bless him for trying, but I always knew. He would say he would have to "make a run" and step out for a while, or I would hear him leave after I went to bed to get up early for work the next morning, but I knew what was going on, and it secretly pissed me off. He would come in and my super sense of smell would be on high alert, and I could smell the delicious foods he had just enjoyed in his clothes. My favorite move by him was his run to get burgers late at night. He crept into his room on the tenth night of fasting and tried to enjoy his sandwich without waking me, but I laid in bed, smelling the air, dreaming of the grease and forbidden calories racing down my throat into my tummy, and I fell asleep thinking I was full. I later found out that Bill tried to turn on the fan and blow the smell out of his window. What happened instead was he blew the smell into my room. Once again, God bless him for trying.

To add to the bad timing of doing the liquid fast, I had to sit through my own team's soccer banquet and not eat. It was heartbreaking to watch everyone enjoying the catered food around me. I kept a smile on my face, and thanked people for the kind comments of me staying strong and being proud of me (I had shared the news with the girls once they noticed me walking around with the plastic cup that came with my package at the games, which meant the parents knew everything by this time) but I wanted to eat. I even started to shake at the banquet due to the lack of food, but I didn't share how I felt with anyone at this important event for my girls. I was sweating, and my hands couldn't stop shaking, and I thought I was going to pass out, but the show had to go on, and I made it through the award presentation. I was so sad, and so wanted the liquid fast to end.

The other terrible side effect of the liquid fast was my development of headaches. It was my number one symptom of withdrawal, and they started on day four. The pulsation on the side of my head was crushing my skull. There was nothing that could stop the pounding in my head, and it went on almost ten days. I placed cold rags on my eyes, I cut the lights off at work during break and when I got home, and I rubbed my temples, but nothing helped, the headache was a part of me.

So I couldn't watch TV due to the commercials, I couldn't concentrate due to my headaches, and I had to deal with my stomach constantly growling at the changes. I can truly say that I was at a new level of miserable.

The last part before surgery was doing one more exam, but this time, it was at the hospital. It was the hospital's way of making sure they had all my information, and to make sure I had been a good girl and completed my pre-surgery diet. My blood pressure was taken again, along with some blood work, and finally, my weight.

I was down to 304. My blood pressure was lower and I was taken off one of my medications. Things were changing.

The diet had taken its effect before surgery, and I had lost some weight. Some people had told me that I looked slimmer, but I didn't believe them until that moment. The liquid diet was one of the hardest things that I had done, and it killed me to know that I had two weeks to go with the same diet. But I had to remember that all of shakes were for my benefit, and it was better to follow the directions of my medical staff. I could do it, even if I were miserable for a short time longer.

SURGERY DAY

It was finally here. After multiple doctor's appointments, pre surgery testing, needles for blood work and protein shakes for weeks, it was finally the day. Amazingly, I had slept well the night before, and woke up nervous, but well rested. I had to do my pre surgery preparation the night before, 24 hours of clear liquids, and a shower with a special substance that would disinfect my body before surgery. I had to shower with the same liquid when I woke up, and I didn't officially get scared until I was in the shower. I had been so confident all the weeks up to this day, but it was officially here, and there was no turning back once I went into the hospital room. I remember my body trembling as I washed with the anti-bacterial soap. I could barely breathe; I was nervous, excited, happy, and wanted to cry all in the same moment. I knew that this was what was best for me, but the uncertainty was killing me inside. I mean, this surgery could go wrong; this could be the last day of my life. I could be making a huge mistake. Every negative scenario was running through my mind, and I was hoping these thoughts would do down the drain with the shower water, and wash away like my hospital soap.

My parents and Bill were going with me to the hospital. There was debate on where I would stay after surgery, but the decision was for me to stay home, and Bill to would take care of me. My mother was very insistent on me staying at her home, but I had a problem with her two babies, Flora and Sterling. When I say her babies, I am talking about her cats. I actually love Flora and Sterling and they were my babies too, but once I moved out I developed an allergy to cats, and they made it hard for me to breathe and I sneezed constantly. My pre-surgery nurse asked about allergies, and I explained the situation, in which she replied, "Jessyca, there is no way you are staying at your Mommy's house. You are going to have four incisions in your stomach, and if you sneeze and pop something, you will be very angry at that decision."

This meant that Bill had to be my caregiver, which, as I mentioned before, was a lot to ask from a best friend, but he agreed to take on the challenge. Bill and my parents were ready to cheer for me.

I slipped on grey sweatpants, a blue homecoming t-shirt, and did a silent prayer while putting on my pink slippers. Bill was ready, and I could tell he was nervous for me, but trying to cover it up. The same worried expression was on my parents' faces when they pulled into the drive way to pick us up. When I think back on it, I think they were more nervous about it than I was.

My medical center is located in heart of Flint, MI, and has one of the most reputable standings in the medical world in bariatric surgery. All of the surgeons had awards and certifications more than a person thinking of this surgery could ask for, but to be honest, I had never used this hospital for anything medical before this. I always lived outside the city, and never used the inner city hospitals, and I had no idea what to expect.

The first positive thing I will say about my hospital is that everyone there is uncontrollably friendly. I am amazed how you walk right through the doors and everyone is smiling and wanting to take care of you. When we walked in and went to the information booth, the woman who greeted us was so loving and took such great care of us. We walked through the winding halls, and I registered at the pre-op desk. The large flock of people in the waiting room made me wide eyed, and the reality of this step officially took over my mind.

"You are going to do this surgery, Jes. It's the right choice. Stay calm, just breathe and give it to God."

There was a moment when I settled in my waiting room chair that I wanted to grab a hold of some one's arm and cuddle against it like a child for comfort, but I resisted. I sat with my mom, and my father and Bill sat across from me. The men did the typical waiting room masculine moves, my father reached for something to read, and Bill looked for a plug for his laptop. My mother sat next to me, with her hands folded in her lap. I think she did this to resist tapping her pretty red nails due to her nervous energy. I found out while waiting that I could only have one person come with me in my prepping room before entering surgery, and I, of course, chose my Mommy. There is nothing like the words of Mom during something that could potential change your life, it was a no brainer choice.

I received an armband with my information, filled out the last stages of paper work, and waited impatiently for my name was called. My surgery was scheduled for 10:30 A.M., and everything seemed to be working like clockwork when they called my name to come back with my mother. I gave my dad a reassuring look, looked at Bill, he gave me a quick wink for good luck, and my mother and I were off for me to be prepped for surgery.

After getting dressed in the "barely covering my body" white gown, they placed the IV in my arm and I was laid down on the hospital gurney in a cold waiting room. My mom was given a seat with me and we waited. And waited more. And more. I waited so long that the nurses had to keep putting warm blankets on me, and they offered my mother something to read and drink. I thought because I was nervous that time was going slowly, but something was wrong, it was way pass 10:30 A.M.

A nurse came by and discussed that there were complications with the surgery before mine, which terrified me because that means that things could go wrong. She assured me that they would come to get me soon, but I ended up waited almost an hour and a half passed my surgery time. During my waiting time the nurses gave more warm blankets, my mom kept my spirits up and I worked on my deep breathing exercises to stay calm. Despite all that support, the nurse had to come and drug me, which I was thankful for because I needed something to take the edge off and help me not panic. They gave me a medicine to just take care of my nerves because they wouldn't give me the heavy drugs until it was time for the actual surgery. Suddenly, a kindly nurse walked into the room, smiled, and said, "Jessyca, it's time to go."

My mom, who worked hard to suppress her worried face, smiled and kissed my forehead. I told her I would see her soon, and there was a click of the wheels being released on my hospital gurney, and I began my transportation to the operating room.

There were two nurses, having small talk pushing me through the crowds of people in the hallway on the way to the room that would change my life. They were very polite, and wanted to make sure I was fine before the big event. Strangely, I was at peace at this moment. It could have been the drugs, or it could have been the fact that I was ready for this. I had accepted that this was the right thing for me, and that I shouldn't worry because I would be fine.

The operating room was so bright and strangely void with color. The walls were the brightest shade of white I had seen, and a saw a table with tools that were going to be used on me, standing in the corner. My heart began to speed up.

I looked around for the doctor, but he had not arrived. One of the nurses must have noticed my expression and said, "The doctor won't be here until you go under, Jessyca. We are here to get you situated and make you comfortable. Don't worry, we are here for you."

I nodded, took a deep breath, and followed the nurse's instructions. I hopped from the gurney I was in onto the operating table. I made myself as comfortable as I could while they adjusted my IV and placed all the surgical supplies around me. I remember a bright light being turned on me. It blinded my vision for a moment, but that light was all I could focus on before my surgery.

"OK, Jessyca. We are going to give you some medicine to knock you out, girl. When you wake up, you will be a new woman! Are you ready?"

My heart was racing rapidly, so much that I could hear its pitter patter thumping against my rib cage. The time was now, there was no turning back. It's now.

"I'm ready. And thank you," was my reply.

I remember a cold rush in my arm. Its icy chill tingled, and I felt it flow through my veins. My body began to feel heavy, and I could feel myself start to fight the sleep. I stared at the light and began to pray. The prayer was one I had said many times before my big day, so that if it were my last words on earth, the wording would be perfect.

Dear Lord,

Thank you for this opportunity and thank you for a new life. Please watch over everyone if I don't wake up and let them know I am happy. Take care of my family, friends, my best friend, and my kids. Let them know I love them for being there. Lord...I'm thankful...Forgive me...I'm scared...

PAIN AND PAMELA

When I came to from the anesthesia there was an older gentleman sitting next to my bed. I blinked several times, trying to wake completely from the medicated haze they had put me under. It felt like I had slept 10 minutes, but it had been a couple hours, and I was in the recovery room. I turned my head to the left and stared at the strange man sitting next to me. He has lost the majority of his hair and had a grey beard. He was reading something when he noticed me start the stir, and placed the book in his lap when I turned my head toward him. He smiled at me, and rested his hands on top of his book.

"Well, hello there, Jessyca. You have decided to join us again. How are you feeling?"

I didn't really think about how I was doing until he asked, but the answer was obvious when I thought about it. Only two words explained the feelings in my abdomen, "tight" and "pain". I felt a tightness I had never felt before, and it felt like someone was stepping on my stomach. There was pain running across the whole midsection of my body, and I could feel the thombing of my body reacting to the surgery. They had done four incisions in my body, with the largest one near my belly button. The pain was everywhere, and I started to panic. I answered the gentlemen who pose the question how I was doing.

"I hurt," was all I said.

"Well, honey, you're gonna hurt. You just had some major surgery. But don't worry, you did wonderfully."

It turned out my surgery went better than expected. It was quick and easy for surgeon and his staff, and they had hopes of me healing quickly. I found this all out the next day, but the man just saying that things went "wonderfully" made me feel much better.

I just wanted to see my family and friend when I came too. I waited a short time and was transported to my room for the night. I had to wait for a while to see anyone because there was testing that needed to be done and more drugs for me to take. I was pretty mellow when my family finally came in.

The first person I saw was my grandmother, Grams Edna. Grams would always come to the hospital for anyone, be it major surgery or a sprained ankle. My uncle, Mark, had brought her to join my parents and Bill in the waiting room. She strolled over and patted my arm, and asked if I was doing alright. I think I replied to her, but then my parents walk in the room, followed by Bill, who smiled at me and settled in the chair straight across from my bed. Everyone was asking questions and making small talk, except for William, he kept staring at something on the other side of the room, then outside the window, then me, and then at the paper. He hated hospitals, and so did my father, who looked equally uneasy while standing in the corner. Dad figured out how to turn the television on for everyone, and showed me how to work the remote. Everyone wanted to make sure I was situated and that I was fine. I found out later that I looked like hell, which might have been the reason everyone was so caring. My torso was bloated, my hair was everywhere, and, in layman's terms, I was borderline high. The one thing I can remember really clear was telling everyone that I was really tired, and they looked tired too and needed to go home and rest.

Everyone came to the bed and said their goodbyes. I turned the TV to World Cup and watched until the medicine sent me to sleep. I woke up a couple hours later, with a nurse saying I had a phone call.

I was so confused. Who would be calling me while I was in the hospital? My parents would contact everyone, so it wasn't family, and Bill was letting all my friends know how I was doing on social media and phone calls. Who could be calling?

I took the phone and listened for the person's voice. "Guuuurl, how you doing up in that hospital after surgery?"

I might have been groggy from the medication, but there was no way I wouldn't know that country twangs from anyone else's dialect. It was Ms. Fantroy.

Sherron worked at my school for a couple years. She was one of the most brutally honest people I had in my life before she moved back South. Her husband was a preacher, and the family was called back South for him to preach the word. Being the good minister's wife, Sherron gathered her things and her beautiful daughters and left my school and me behind. We had talked briefly about me having surgery (I didn't share the news with too many people due to me being such a private person), but I didn't expect her to call the hospital with greetings. God sends you blessings when you need them, and hearing Sherron's country voice was a blessing indeed.

Sherron Fantroy asked me how I was doing and demanded to know how the people were treating me. Despite my stomach hurting I giggled heavily at her silly questions and stories about the kids. She was a ray of light for me on this long, healing evening, and I still don't have the words to express my gratitude for her taking time to look up the hospital number and to call me during her busy day. She closed the conversation with, "Alright, guuuurl. I'm not playing with you about taking it easy. Do what they say and don't be stubborn. I am praying for you and love ya, guuuurl." I said I loved Sherron back.

The most interesting thing of the night was my roommate, Pamela. I didn't even realize she was there for a long time until I heard a conversation about her in the hall. Pam had the same surgery that I did, and actually she had her surgery before I did. I later that evening found out that the reason my surgery started so late was because of Pam. I didn't see her the first part of the night, but I knew she was there, because she kept moaning, loudly. She had been given a morphine pump for her pain, which they didn't even offer to me. I was in pain, but not to the point that I needed to have nonstop medication. Pam was a difficult patient for the nurses, and she constantly pushed the button for assistance, begging for more medication. She had used a full day's medicine in her morphine pump in just four hours, and the hospital refused to give her anything else. She made noises all through the night, and I didn't understand why she was in so much pain when she had the same procedure I did. At one point, she started a conversation with me. I still hadn't seen her; the curtain was drawn so we could have "privacy".

In the middle of one of her late night moaning sessions is when she started a conversation with me. She asked me my name and which surgery I had. She then ask me what doctor and what time it was scheduled, which was when I discovered that she was actually the surgery before mine. I next found out why her surgery took so long. She was suspiciously inquisitive.

"Did you cheat on your pre surgery diet?" she whispered.

I didn't even think of playing around with the diet. My life would be on the line if I screwed up, at least that was the way I felt. To be honest with you, the shakes do fill you up for quite a few hours. I didn't even think of cheating, although I had some people do some serious temptation toward me to not follow the doctor's orders. Despite my feelings of despair, I followed the doctor's orders.

"No, I didn't cheat on the diet. Did you?"

The answer Pam had for me was quite surprising, and she was paying a heavy price for her weakness in her diet. The reason why she was in so much pain was because she did not following the directions. Pam liked pizza rolls.

This woman started to explain to me that she chose to eat pizza rolls the day before surgery. And she decided to indulge in thin sliced ham. Pam was paying the price because since her stomach wasn't empty during the time of surgery, she had to have all the bad foods pumped out of her stomach before even having the surgery. It is explained to anyone that eating the night before could lead to complications that could result in death. I was horrified that this woman chose pizza rolls over her health and she could have killed herself. That was why she was moaning, the reason she was in extreme pain, and it was hard to pity her situation, but remember that food addiction can have a powerful hold on its victims.

Food is a weakness for anyone who has bariatric surgery, but if you can't commit to the pre-surgery diet plan, then you don't need to do the surgery, period. Food is not worth dying for, and the mental commitment is just as important as the physical commitment. To sum things up, Pam was a mess in many ways.

This woman made noises all night, and you could hear her constantly jabbing the morphine drip button. My night was spent listening to her beg for medicine, and hitting the emergency light for the nurses. You could see their annoyance out in the hallway with Pam because of her poor choices, and in the middle of this nonsense I decided I would do whatever the doctors and nurses said to do to get out of that hospital room as soon as possible in the morning.

The main nurse that I can remember through this whole ordeal turned out to know someone from my past. She was the mom of a guy I went to high school with, and she was wonderful. She was like a family member when she took care of me in the middle of the night. She gave me medicine, she told me stories, and she made sure that I followed all the directions the doctor had laid out for me. She was a God sent woman, and I appreciated her.

Also in the middle of the night I went for my first walk after surgery with one of the third shift nurses. It was essential to show that you could walk as progress to be released. I was asked to walk as soon as I could due to me having a blood clot six years before, because many people developed Deep Vein Thrombosis right after surgery. I walked the entire fourth floor with my nurse, and she cheered each step I took. She gave me encouraging words and told me that if I could keep down the liquids they gave me in the morning and pass a medical test, I would be released. That excited me more than you can imagine, and I lay to rest with a smile on my face. I was going home tomorrow.

KEEP ON LOVING YOU!

I woke the next morning feeling less sore. I still couldn't bend really well, but I did have the ability to reach for the remote with no problem. I stared at the morning sunrise and enjoyed that this was the first complete day of my new life. I felt a new sense of happiness that I didn't change my mind about completing the surgery, but deep down in my soul, I was still slightly terrified of what my new life would entail.

The new shift nurse came in and checked my vitals and said with a happy face, "Jessyca, we are going to send you for some test and then try and get some liquids in you. Keep them down, and you get to go home!"

I had done everything they asked and was praying to go home from the hospital. After a couple hours I was sent for testing. The test was simple: drink a cloudy liquid and let them take x-rays to make sure there wasn't any leakage in my new banded belly. Everything came back positive with my testing, and I was brought back to my room.

When I came back to the room, I finally had a chance to look at my wailing hospital room mate.

I will share with you that at pre-surgery testing, I weighed in at 318 pounds, which made me cry in the car. As I said earlier, I am, as declared by our society, a "thick" built girl, and when I say that number to people they are astonished I carried that much weight on my body. I also should share that I shouldn't react when seeing someone bigger than me, but at this time, I regrettably have to share that I did indeed react to the sight of Pamela.

Pam was almost double my size.

Pam was a massive woman, and she looked in poor shape. I was so surprised that a woman that size would have the same surgery that I did. I am not saying that my reaction was fair, but I have to be honest about what I thought when I saw her. She was sprawled across the bed, with morphine button still in her hand, and oxygen attached to her nose. If you were to see the two of us, a person would never guess we had the same surgery. She was still moaning, with her head tilted towards the heavens. My sister would say that the woman was "a hot mess."

I went to the restroom (which was another requirement for me to go home) and then slowly eased myself back on my hospital bed. A nurse came in with a tray of different liquids that I needed to try. I had a bowl of chicken broth, apple juice, a small protein shake, and some gelatin. It was my job to drink what I could and to keep it down. Everything was in mini size, which I learned would be my food quantity for the rest of my life.

Lesson number one of drinking after surgery is to "Sip! Sip! Sip!" When you become banded, you give up the ability to "gulp" things down. You do baby sips of your fluids, because if you don't, it will shoot back up. The nurses stated for me to just sip and they would check on me, and to take my time.

I will never forget the first sip. I felt it and I knew things were different. There was a strange tightness in my belly, and it reacted oddly toward the first liquid that I took in my body. I sat there and concentrated on the feel of the ice water trickling down through my stomach. This was odd, and I knew I had some new things to learn about my new "GB" life.

Nurses cheered my sipping, and they took out my IV. My father and Bill were coming to get me, and I smiled while enjoying my Strawberry protein shake while watching World Cup Soccer. I didn't finish my items on my tray, and it turns out I wasn't supposed to get everything down. Time passed quickly, and I suddenly saw my father in the doorway.

Dad walked by and didn't see my hospital roommate due to walking directly to me to see how I was doing. Bill, on the other hand, walked in, looked at Pam, looked at me, looked at Pam again with wide eyes, then at the wall, and then rushed to the chair. Bill shared with me later that he saw that Pam weighed over 550 pounds, and her physical status terrified him. We sat and visited for a while, waiting for the clearance papers, when I heard the nurses trying to convince Pam to drink her liquids. She refused.

"Pam, you aren't leaving the hospital if you don't prove you are fit to do so. You have to drink the liquids. We can't even give you anymore medicine until you show an effort to follow directions. Please drink."

Pam laid there and moaned louder, and Bill's eyes grew larger. My father whispered to me, asking what surgery Pam had. I (in hushed tones) explained the details of the night with her, and he shook his head in horror. I then told Bill of my nightly adventures and he tucked his chin into his chest and chuckled under his breath. As I was sharing the details of the Pam's saga with the boys, she received visitors, who practically begged her to drink, but she continued to refuse. My father, Bill, and I actually gave up talking so we could listen to "The Adventures of Pam". At one point, her husband's phone rang, and the three of us almost burst into laughter. It was one of the most well-known power ballads of all time.

Was I really hearing REO in my hospital room? It took all Bill and Dad had not to burst out laughing at the ring tone, especially with her husband persistently trying to get Pam to drink the fluids. It seemed just so perfect for that song to play at that time, and whenever I hear it, I think of Pam and her husband. Even with the charming ring tone, and all the begging from her man, there was no changing Pam's mind, and people gave up trying to convince her to do the right thing.

The papers came and I signed out with joy. I had already changed (with the help of my nurses) before the boys came, and the struggle to leave began. I needed help to put on my Snoopy Slippers, help to ease into the wheelchair, help getting wheeled down to the elevator, help to get out the wheelchair and to ease into the car. I hope you see the emphasis on the repetitive use of the word, "help." Anyone who has this surgery done will need lots of the "h" word, for quite a long time. It's amazing how much you use your abdomen area and you take it for granted that it would always be there to work for you.

The hospital supplied me with a huge elastic band that I had to wear around of abdomen for two weeks. The only time I didn't have to wear it was when I was taking a shower or sleeping, but the rest of the time, it was my healthy corset. I also left with an ice pack, which I clung to when I got into the car. The nurse smiled and said "Good Luck" while Bill was placing me in the car, and away we went.

When my father pulled up my house, I was excited to see the doorway, but scared to get out the car due to the pain. Bill's loyalty to me was in overdrive starting this day, and he immediately hopped out the car, open the car door for me like a true gentleman, helped me ease slowly out of the front seat, and took my arm to bring me inside. He was with me every step toward the big, red couch that my elementary buddy Kimmy gave me before surgery, and he eased me down gently on its right corner with three of my pillows.

That short trip made me very tired, and very sore. My father took the script for my prescriptions that the nurse handed him as we walked out the hospital to the local drug store because my body was thumping from the pain, and I needed the meds. Bill brought me a large ice water and set it on the table, and sat across from me. Any movement I made, he jumped, and his concern was heartwarming. My mother was over my house, doing what mother's do with making everything in the house easily accessible. My mother is amazing in times like these, and I hope to have the skills that she does when I get older. The cups were on the cabinet so I didn't have to reach for them, the bathroom had everything laid out for me, and she did busy talk to keep me occupied. She was doing the "motherly love" job wonderfully, and I appreciated all the efforts that people were doing to make me comfortable.

I was home.

DID MY STOMACH JUST GROWL?

My doctor required for me to do two more weeks of protein shakes before having any kind of solid food. The first week home was tough, not because I wanted to eat, but because I couldn't drink all that the doctors wanted me to drink. They still wanted to me drink five shakes a day, plus at least 48-64 ounces of water. I felt that this task was nearly impossible, but I tried my best to follow the medical professionals' demands. I don't think I did the five shakes any of those days because my belly would get so full, and the closest I came to was four in one day. Many times I would gag on trying to do all the shakes, and the last thing I wanted to do was puke after having this surgery. I was told that if I got sick I could make the band slip or pop my stitches, and with the pain I was experiencing, that was not an option.

During the healing process I had to wear a giant, girdle like support band around my torso that I talked about earlier, which also was uncomfortable at times. It would pinch when I would be sitting on the couch and would roll up at times, which required me to do one thing I couldn't stand during my first week at home, stand up. I couldn't stand in the first week of recovery without someone's help, and the energy to stand and fix that girdle was a pain in more ways than one. I slept on the couch the first two weeks of recovery in an upright position due to trying to heal, and all that time I was so uncomfortable.

I kept following rule number 1, "Sip! Sip! Sip!" I was required to walk every couple hours so that I didn't develop another blood clot, and that was quite difficult. It was Bill's job to force me to walk, and to listen to me complain and beg to stay seated on the couch.

He would listen to my whining for a short time and then would demand me to "get my ass up", which I always did.

It hurt so bad to stand up. All those muscles that the surgeon had to go through to get to my stomach had taken a major beating, and to walk the first couple days was dreadful. The support band that I had to wear each day did help to keep my abdomen secure, but the incisions were distressing. But I walked like I needed to, holding on to someone's arm or to the wall, and as the days passed, the walking moved from baby steps to steps of confidence on my own. The walking began to get easier.

The shakes started to become more manageable, and the swelling of my belly started to ease. After the first week, I finally took the bold step of really looking at the incisions. Two of the scars were pretty small, one medium sized, but I stared at the largest one. This one was near my belly button, and was quite a bit puffier than the others. I later found out that this incision was the one that they slid the device in with. It wasn't grossly large, but it did stand out more than the rest. I also found out that if you push on the right spot of this incision, you can feel the band's port, which I use to gross people out for my own amusement.

I grabbed my phone and started to take pictures of my belly. I wanted a reminder of the process that I went through to become healthier. I stared at the pictures; it wasn't that bad from the camera lens's viewpoint. Yes, I was swollen, but it wasn't like I had a scar that ran all the way down my midsection. There was some redness around the cuts, but nothing too alarming, but the swelling did make my stomach look like a caramel colored hill due to its roundness.

In the middle of the second week of healing, a strange event happened. My stomach growled. I felt like a child discovering a new function of the body when it happened, because I quickly looked down and grabbed my sides. I even said aloud, "Did my stomach just growl?" and then I just laughed. It had finally become angry with the shakes, and the lack of chewing delicious food. It had become irate at the demands of just liquid. It wanted real food and it wanted it now!

I only had a couple more days until I visited the doctor and started stage two of my food phase, but my stomach wasn't agreeing with the schedule. It wanted pizza, Chinese food, ice cream, and all the things I knew I couldn't have. It became a battle of mental strength over hunger. My stomach growled for two whole days, giving me echoing reminders that I was hungry.

Despite the anger of my tummy, my will power won every time. I drank water, sipped on shakes, and ate frozen sugar-free treats. I started to count the days until I had the chance of eating real food, and begin to notice my face getting even thinner. My tummy would just have to be patient, and real food would make its appearance when it needed to.

FAT FLASHBACK
HIGH SCHOOL NOTE WRITING

It is the tradition of high schoolers to get excited about dances. It was a time to dress up, be pretty, take pictures and have unbelievable experiences that you bragged about with your girlfriends after an enchanted evening filled with romance. At least, this is what they tell young girls to be ready to experience. I can say that I did not have that experience with dances, and despite some good memories, the majority of the bad outcomes came from me being fat.

I didn't even go to high school dances until senior year. I felt that it was too much of a burden on my family, and for someone to walk up and ask me to go to a dance was nearly impossible. I don't want you to think that I was an unliked in high school. Actually, I was quite the opposite. I was an athlete, well liked, and, as people have told me over the years, one of the girls that everyone knew. I don't have many tales of people being cruel to me in high school, and I had an enjoyable time during that period. I think that is part of the reason that I insisted on teaching older children when I made the decision to focus my career on education. But high school dances were a completely different story.

I made the decision to take control of my senior year and to attend dances like most children my age. My independent stage kicked in at the beginning of senior year, and I decided not to wait on some guy to ask me to dances, I would choose the man to take me to dances.

I had a crush on a kid and I decided to do the typical 90s way of asking him to a dance. I wrote him a note. This is a lost art now with the advancements of technology and texting, but those who spent hours writing the right words to boys during the times before cell phones completely understand the efforts that are needed to perform this act. I sat for hours writing that note, and trying to get my point across of how great it would be for us to have fun at the dance.

I folded it up perfectly and passed the note to him in the hall. I breathed a sigh of relief that I was strong enough to be able to write and deliver the letter. It was a major accomplishment in my self-esteem and I was happy all day for finding my inner warrior that was fighting for my right to be like everyone else.

My happiness carried me through the school day and on the car ride home with my friend, Sarah. It lasted a couple hours until my friend Lynnea called. She didn't want to tell me what had happened on the bus, but she said that she was my friend and had to share the news. I was the topic of discussion with my crush and another boy that I thought I was friends with. They were laughing hysterically at my note, and even more so that I could dare to think of asking him to the dance. Every reference was toward my weight, and how funny I would look in a dress. They did it the whole bus ride home, and everyone overheard them.

I was devastated that I was teased and unable to defend myself from the attacks. All those people will be laughing at me the next day at school. I started to cry, and Lynnea kept saying, "I'm so sorry, Jes" over and over. The dream of the dance night fantasy was ruined.

Now, a weak woman would have just folded up in a corner and said, "I'm never going to dances ever again" but like I stated earlier, this was when the "warrior" side officially came to be. This fat girl would not lose on this situation, and I was going to win! I cried a little longer, and I sat down and wrote another letter. This one didn't take multiple drafts, it was a one time letter, and it was short and to the point. I folded it up with care, just like the first note, and placed it in my backpack.

The next day I went about my business like things were normal. I didn't care if people were gossiping about me nor had pity on me for the conversation they heard on the bus. I wasn't worried, because I knew that I was going to be alright. I held my head high, and acted like nothing could affect me.

I found the guy, walked up to him, and smiled. He smiled back like he was happy to see me, and that he wasn't the boy who was completely disrespecting me less than 24 hours before. I told him I had a note for him, and placed it gently in my hand. I walked away with a smile on my face, and I never gave him a second thought when it came to the romance department.

I know what the question is. "What did you put in the letter?"

It's simple. I cursed him out. I called him dirty and disrespectful. I told him he would regret missing out on the opportunity of going to the dance with the hottest fat chick that would be there. Finally, I ended it with a "and if I hear of you talking badly about me again, I will personally fuck you up."

You have to remember that I was a teenage girl, and the reply would come across as childish, but I promise you that I would still say this to him, in this same manner, today. I was sick of people disrespecting me about my weight, and I wasn't going to be that girl who wallowed in pity. Oh no, I would dare someone to say something to me about that, and they needed to be ready for my reaction. The wall was officially up with boys, which has led to the even bigger wall with men about my weight later on in my life

Here's the funny aspect of this fat flashback:

Years later I went to my ten year reunion. I was hanging out with one of my old school friends when he came walking in, greeting everyone. He went to my friend, hugged her and asked about her life, and looked over and smiled. He asked her, "Who is your friend, or is this your relative?" My friend looked at me, then looked at him, and with bewilderment said, "Boy, you don't recognize Jes when you see her?"

He was dumbfounded on how much I had changed, and greeted me with such happiness. He wanted to know everything, and was so glad to see me that he offered to buy me drinks. I, of course, refused, and told him about my wonderful life, and made sure to look him in the eyes and shine my beautiful white teeth. I leaned in and rested my chest on my arms so that he could she how ample I was. I was enjoying listening to his story about not finishing college, and still staying in the same house that he was in when he turned me down in high school 10 years before. We talked often during the night, and he even hugged me when I decided to leave. I smiled in his face and made sure to swish my hips as I left. As I got to the door, I whispered the words "Fuck You" and smiled as I entered the early fall air. I was childish once again, and again I didn't feel bad about it.

WASTING AWAY

The first steps of new food were pretty boring foods, but if you had been like me and had shakes for a month, you would have thought that those simple foods were a gourmet meal. I was able to eat wheat crackers with low salt, boiled eggs, small amounts of condiments, and salsa. I drank chicken broth and worked my way up to mashed potatoes. All the foods were very bland and with little to no seasoning, but it wasn't another shake and that was fine with me. I took a new stage of eating more solid foods every two weeks, and I would grow impatient waiting for the time period to end so that I could try something new. But I was able to introduce more foods, and I started to adjust to the new life. When I ate, I could feel the food working down, and it was disturbing for a while, but I got used to it. I also started to count each time I chewed my food. Banded patients are asked to chew their food 25-30 times before swallowing it, which has led to by OCD way of enjoying my food now. Every time I put any food in my mouth, I am secretly chewing to a countdown, and I won't swallow until I reach 30 due to the fear of food getting stuck. The shakes went away, but the amount of water did not. Bottled water became my friend, and I took it with me everywhere, and I adjusted to drinking low calorie drinks for my enjoyment. I discovered that nutra-sweet was not a tool of the devil, and that I could drink it with a smile on my face. I was adjusting well, and didn't miss the old life too much.

One of my biggest excitements was receiving permission to exercise. I still needed to be very careful with my mid-section, but I received permission to begin working out lightly by doing activities like walking and light lifting. I had prepared myself to start a workout regime with my new toy, the Wii Fit. I bought the Wii

Fit from former co-workers, wife, a pleasant woman named Maria. Little does she know the idea of me using this item lead me to my new life of fitness. She said she never used it and thought that it would help me to get back into the swing of things in working out. I bought it from her at a discounted price, and laid it in the corner of the living room until I received permission to give it a try.

This wonderful workout device filled an hour of my day during to healing process. Sometimes I could do the whole hour, sometimes my body died after 30 minutes, but I made sure to use it almost every day if my body would let me. It kept track of my weight, and my balance, and gave me a variety of exercises that I could do each day.

I was shocked when I weighed myself for the first time on the game. Before surgery, I was 318, when I weighed in I was 298! I had lost pounds before surgery due to the shake diet, but slowly the excess weight was starting to melt away. My heart raced at the fact that this band was really working, and my mind flooded with the thoughts that I could lose more weight if I make sure to work out. The Wii Fit would be my tool for success, and I would use it to get myself back on track.

And I did. I used that thing day in and day out, and started to take walks down the street and back. I stuck to my commitment to work hard to get my life on a healthier path. Some days, my body was so heavy and I couldn't work out, but the next day, I made sure to drag myself to do something to make myself fit. When I finished my workout, I was so tired. I would think of the days in high school where I played games and practiced for hours, but that was the younger me, and that energy just wasn't with me at this point in my life. I sweated like crazy when I worked out, and sometimes needed to take breaks for water because I felt like passing out, but I made sure to keep going because it was best for me.

My favorite workout on the Wii Fit was boxing. It started with a couple minutes and then me stopping because my body was crying out the phrase, "Are you crazy" but I slowly increased my time. I punched the air with a vengeance, and thought about all the things that made me angry and put on the weight that almost destroyed me. In my mind, I yelled at the items that were almost my demise.

"Take that birth control meds that made me gain weight!"

"And that hit was for you, the blood clot that almost killed me!"

"This hit is for you, boys who have dogged me out in my life!"

"Screw all of you!!!"

I figured that mentally screaming at all my hardships would give me the willpower to continue, and it did.

The weight slowly started to come off, but I of course didn't notice it. When you have been physically fat for as long as I was, you can look in the mirror every day and still see the same person day after day, even if you are losing the weight. Everyone around me noticed before I did. My parents noticed. My best friend noticed. But I noticed nothing in the beginning stages. To me, I was still fat.

I didn't really accept that I was losing weight until a friend from work told me. I was working summer school to earn some extra money when I had a talk with my friend and co-worker, Mike. We were hired the same day at our school district, and I can say that he is one of the best and most honest teachers I know. Mike, better known as "Stew" was working summer school too, and was one of the four people who saw my process throughout the summer and knew that I had done the surgery.

Stew and I were having one of our many conversations when he stopped and looked at me.

"How are you feeling, Jes?"

I paused and I told him I was feeling pretty good. He asked if I were healing alright and how I was adjusting, and I answered him casually, like I always did. Stew sat and listened to my tales of starting to work out and eating new foods.

"You've definitely lost weight, Jes. I can see it. You look good."

I remembered blinking hard that Stew had given me a compliment. I wasn't use to receiving praise about my weight, and him saying such kind words startled me. I said a quick "thanks" to Stew and headed home. I went to my room, shut the door, and looked at myself in the mirror.

I realized that I had lost weight. My clothes were loose, and my face was thinner. It was slowly coming off and I hadn't really realized it. Why didn't I see it before?

Another group that pointed out that I was wasting away was my grandparents, Burnie and Evon. The main compliment came from Grandpa Evon that took me by surprise. Grandpa was much like my father, except for the silent part. He was a man with an opinion, always. He had his view and he was going to tell you about his view. He would listen to your view, but he would make sure to show a contradiction to your point in a heartbeat. I know that my competitive edge comes from him, and he would be brutally honest on how I looked.

My grandmother is a gentle woman, and I get my height from her. She is actually shorter than me, and stands about 5'1" but I laughed when she first saw me. She came over and patted my stomach, then my hips, and then my butt.

"You've lost a little something, gal," was her joking expression.

My grandfather gave me look over, and put his mighty hands on his hips.

"Granddaughter, you keep this up and I won't be able to see you. That weight is just wasting away!" Grandpa approved of the changes.

After speaking to Stew and my grandparents, I came to the realization that the physical change in me would be faster than the psychological side of me. I would change my physical appearance way faster than my mental state. I had to start thinking thinner, thinking healthier, thinking like a new me. That would be the toughest part of this journey, and if I didn't start thinking thinner, I would never be happy. I smiled at the reflection that showed in the mirror. I was changing, but I had a long way to go physically and mentally to be satisfied with myself.

THE SOCIAL NETWORK

I have found social media to be another wonderful friend of mine during making myself new. I didn't post for a while about the surgery, but when you have tons of free time during the summer, you can use social networking as a tool of spreading your story to others. I began to post about my new life on social media to my friends, and they gave me the strength to work hard to become a more complete person.

I started to receive messages from friends from work, friends from high school, and family that I couldn't visit during this time. I would post about the good and the bad, and my emotions during this time. My first post was the night before going into the hospital for surgery, and people were so kind with sending me well wishes for a successful recovery. I saved some of my friends messages that made me smile when I spent those healing weeks on the couch, and I go back and read them when I am not doing well emotionally. I had so many positive people around me on social media, and it made me feel better.

Oddly enough, I didn't mind posting messages and status updates, but I did mind posting pictures. For months, I refused to post a picture. People would write and request me to send them a picture, but I would make up excuses to why I couldn't send them a picture or post it on my wall. I didn't want people thinking negatively, or thinking that I didn't change at all and was still fat. I wouldn't post a picture for anyone, until my friend Kim insisted.

Kim and I have been close since Dye Elementary, and she is one of my true friends. I know in our society we use the term friends loosely, but Kim is the definition of the word "friend". She will forever be my favorite girl. She lives far away from me, but I know she will drop everything for me if I called with trouble, and I would do the same.

Kim wrote me a message, telling me to stop being dumb and to post a picture. She asked me what I was waiting for and to stop hiding from people. I rolled my eyes at her comments and chuckled, but to make her happy I posted a picture.

I sometimes think that Kim making me post started a new obsession with me (which isn't the first time she had done this over the years), but I post pictures all the time now. It forces me to look at myself, and to compare the past to the present. Looking at pictures keeps me on my toes, and keeps me strong and focused on living a healthier lifestyle. My postings of pictures lead to me posting pictures on my fridge for inspiration. I have a soccer picture of me at 318 on my fridge that I refuse to take down, and other pictures that show my progression in weight loss.

I learned that you can't lose weight without examine yourself. You have to look at the old pictures that make you cringe, you have to take lots of pictures during your progress to stay focused, and you have to accept that it is a slow and long progress.

Once again, I focus on is my main area, my face. Not for the change in its size, but my happiness in pictures now. The smile in the latest pictures is genuine, and I am happy to pose in front of a camera. I am going to keep posting more pictures on social media and adding more supportive fans.

TIME FOR A TIGHTENING

One of the most common questions I receive from curious supporters is, "How does the doctor tighten the band?" When I answer this question, I can always count on the same response, a person shrieking back in horror. I guess I would do the same thing if I didn't go through the experience myself.

I had been back to the hospital a couple times before my first "fill." I had an appointment two weeks after surgery to learn about the different phases of food, and to have my incisions checked. Those visits were more like taking food training classes, and I was placed in a room with ten other people who had gone through the surgery around the same week that I had.

One girl in the room actually had her surgery the same day I had mine, and we had run into one another the following day in the X-ray department. We did small talk about how things had gone, and joked about how we were sick of shakes and ready for "real food". The group learned of the different stages of food that we would go through, and how to keep ourselves out of harm's way with our new tummies.

One thing that people take advantage of in our society is the variety of food choices one can have for a day. I grew excited at each food stage after the shakes. Stage one after shakes was protein based foods and soft foods. I was allowed to eat oatmeal with no sugar (which I did one time due to it being disgusting to me). I ate lots of yogurt, and hummus each day. There was apple sauce, hard-boiled eggs, and a development for the love of pita chips and wheat crackers. Lastly, was my favorite of the foods, refried beans with a hint of salsa.

I ate refried beans like they were going out of style in that food stage. My tongue's taste buds celebrated with the taste of this Mexican side dish, and my jaw chewed away at its thick texture. It still is one of my favorite foods after being banded, and there were no issues of eating this, and the other foods, without any digestive issues.

The day before my band tightening I went out with The Spice Girls for a birthday party. The Spice Girls are better known as the English Department of CA, and were my closest friends at work. We gave ourselves the nick name of The Spice Girls after one of our many adventures throughout the school year. Each girl had a role in our group and had a name that fit each personality.

Katherine is better known as Posh Spice, due to her addiction to the fashion world. Posh can tell you what is "in" and what is "out" with your outfits and you would never catch her in school attire that did not make a statement. Katherine always taught in high heels, even while pregnant with her children, and always was a diva and a half.

Carrie is Baby Spice because she is the youngest and the cutest of the crew. She is not a baby in her actions or behavior. To be honest, she is one of the more mature ones in her wisdom inside and outside work, but she is the one that everyone finds adorable.

Judy, the matriarch of the group, was Shakespeare Spice, due to her plethora of intelligence in everything! She would give words of wisdom in times of trouble, and would be there if you were an emotional wreck. Judy was, and will always be the one I run to first, because she always knows what to say.

The most important Spice Girl to me was my neighbor and working best friend, Vera. Instead of making reference to Vera in Spice Girl lingo, I call her my own pet name, V-Boo, and I, in turn, was called J-Boo, by my elbow buddy. Vera is the main person that I love and adore at work, and we are like sisters. We call one another, we text like children, we have secret jokes and pick on one another during lunch. People don't know how to take us, but I couldn't make it through work without my beloved V-Boo. I actually told Vera about my surgery before anyone else at work, and she was one of a small group of people that I spoke to before coming back to work with the new me.

There were other girls of the English Department with fun and entertaining Spice Girl names and we are the divas of the school.

I hadn't seen the crew all summer due to taking care of myself, but I felt good enough to hang out with the posse for a birthday party. It was Baby and Yoga (Mandy) Spice's birthday celebration, and even though I could not have the food and drinking fun like the others, I needed to get out of the house and become social again.

The party was fitting for Yoga Spice's birthday, because Mandy was the high class party animal of the group, so it was only right that the party be at a winery. When I arrived, the girls had already sampled many different styles of Michigan wines, and were in a relaxed and jovial mood. Others from different departments had joined in the celebration and everyone was surprised to see me.

There were compliments, hugs, and words of support as I found a place at the table, and quickly the conversation turned toward my health and my new changes. I answered questions as quickly as I could, because I didn't want to be the center of attention at someone else's party. Girls asked questions and I answered them while they brought out trays of sample glasses of more wine for the patrons to enjoy.

This was the first time that I felt out of place at a gathering. The table was covered with delicious cheeses and desserts, and the aroma of the sweet wine filled the air, and I couldn't enjoy any of it. I felt somewhat saddened by this party, because I officially knew that I had made a major change, and I could not go back to the old me in eating. Everyone else sampled foods and drank merrily, and I sat there sipping on a glass of ice water. There would be many more gatherings like this, and that feeling always came back, that feeling of sadness and agony that I couldn't be like everyone else.

Sarah, a friend from the history department, was the one to ask the classic question about filling the band, and I shared that I would be getting filled the following day. Amber, a Spice Girl member that had the same surgery as I a year before, decided that this was the time to tell me of how painful the fill would be. She went into grim detail of her first fill, and the pain that jetted through her body in the process.

I was alarmed at the information, and other members of the party worked on reassuring me that everything would be alright. I thought about my fill throughout the rest of the party, even when we moved to another location to continue the celebration.

"Would I regret having the band put in? Will it hurt me to have it filled? Is this all worth the hassle?"

I actually left the party early because I couldn't focus on the fun times had by all the members of the party. I kept thinking about the doctor's visit and how it would feel to get the band tightened for the first time. The wise one, Shakespeare Spice, noticed my distress and called me to the other end of the table at the Mexican cantina that we landed at for the last location of the night during the party. She told me not to worry, and Judy was never wrong with her advice.

I didn't sleep well that night. I was tense, and my mind could not rest at the thought of something painful coming after healing from my surgery. I rose that morning and did as instructed by the bariatric center: something light to eat an hour before the appointment and to drink water for good hydration.

I was called back rather quickly, and a medical assistant did the standard procedure of my temperature and my blood pressure. My blood pressure had gone down a decent amount since getting the surgery, and the assistant cheered me for doing well. My weight was down even more and I had hit the 30 pounds lost mark. Once again, I was cheered for my efforts. The assistant stated that the nurse would be in to see me, and my nervousness came back.

The wait for the nurse felt like an eternity. I checked my social networks in my phone, I flipped through the pages of a magazine, and I daydreamed of the fill and the pain that came with the procedure. Suddenly, there was a knock at the door, and the nurse arrived.

The nurse was pleasant, and she asked important questions about my eating habits and vitamin intake. She gave me directions on foods in the next stage, and said that it was time to do the fill. Out on the cabinet were two syringes, cotton swabs, adhesive bandages, and rubber gloves.

I was placed on an elevating table for my band fill, and the nurse made sure to talk me through each step.

The first part of the fill requires the nurse to find the port. The port is a small circle that is located near your bellybutton. During my first fill my port was easy to find, and it was located in the middle of my largest incision scar on my stomach. I sometimes have people feel my port for entertainment. I will rub my belly to find the device, and then have people play with it like a Halloween attraction. I always giggle at people jumping back in horror of the port, and the amazement that I have a foreign device in my body. The nurse examined my scars before finding the port with ease, and then she explained the next step.

With her right hand, the nurse leaned over for the first needle. The first syringe was used to numb the area of my stomach where the port of was found. The shot felt similar to getting a shot while when getting a tooth filled. There was a quick sting from the needle, but nothing that I needed to scream about in agonizing pain. The nurse waited for the medicine to take effect, and we made small talk about me getting ready to return to work, and the changes I had gone through the last couple months.

Next came the actual filling of the band. The nurse explained that the second needle would be inserted into the port, and she would do two things. Step one was to see how much saline was actually in the band. My stomach was numb in the correct location, and she gently inserted the needle into the port. I could feel the needle pressing into my belly, but it didn't hurt like I was told at the party. There was a pressure, an odd pressure, that made me crease my brow not in tremendous pain that I was expecting, but because I felt like someone was stepping on my stomach. During the procedure, the nurse stated that my band was perfect in its functioning, and that she would give me a small fill to see how my body reacted to the newness of the tightened band.

I felt the band deflate and then inflate with the increase of the saline solution, and my stomach did a jump, like a muscle spasm. The process was rather quick, the pain was minimal, and the nurse said that I was done and did a great job.

I always want to embellish the process when people ask about the filling of the band. People assume that my midsection is opened up in a surgery room, and that I return from the operating room, writhing in pain, and in complete agony, but I wasn't and the process was rather simple with limited discomfort. The last thing that was asked from me was to drink water to make sure the band was not too tight. I drank half a glass, and felt perfectly fine after the first procedure. The only medical item I walked out of the center with was a small bandage on my stomach.

After getting the band filled, I had to stay on a liquid and soft food diet for 24 hours. I drank chicken broth and sipped on low calorie drinks. For dinner, I had gelatin, and for breakfast I had pudding. The process of the first fill was not as scary as it had been portrayed, at least, not in my experience.

REAL TEMPTATION

The summer was near an end and it was time to head back to school. I had been banded for a little over two months and other than The Spice Girls party and summer school, I had basically been in hiding. I had to prepare to head back to the daily grind of teaching for yet another school year. I had lost some weight, and needed to buy new clothes.

Shopping for big women is not the same as anyone else. I know that everyone has their struggles with their figure, but the process of selecting clothes for a fat person is a completely different chore. One of the biggest fashion no-no's in my opinion are big girls thinking that just because it is made in their size that it will look good on them. For example, skinny jeans on plus size women. Of course they make them in larger sizes due to making sure to supply a fashionable trend for all markets, but that does not mean that all big girls should put them on. They make some of us look funny, and over exaggerate our hips, our thighs, and our butts, especially if the pants ride low. Women that are big and fashion conscious should be aware of the evils of skinny jeans, they are a tool to make some of us to look foolish.

Plus size women have to try on everything and get hustled for more money. We pay more since there is more cloth needed to make our items, so it is our responsibility to make sure that we are getting more out of our dollars in our fashion. You have to try on everything, and that, in my opinion, is quite annoying.

One of my many hang-ups in shopping is fitting rooms. I hate fitting rooms with a passion. The idea of many people stripping down in a room to slide on clothes creeps me out, and I don't know why. Previously, I would prefer to buy the clothes, try them on at home, and bring them back if they don't work, but you can't do that when you get banded. The size you wear at one store might not work at the next, and you have to try on everything! I had slowly started to get over my phobia of changing rooms, but not completely. I still don't like to sit down on the little stoops they have in there, someone else's butt might have been there, but that is my personal issue (I blame this on the OCD too).

I made my first journey out to buy a couple outfits for the new school year. I figured I only needed a couple pair of black pants, three shirts, and a pair of jeans. I didn't want to spend much due to the hopes that I wouldn't be able to fit them in a couple months, and I planned on keeping my wardroom very basic.

I went into the store and started to look on the clearance rack to find a couple items and realized I had no idea what size I was at this point. The last thing I wanted to do was spend hours in the grossness known as a dressing room, so I had to ask for assistance for some measurements.

There was one girl at this particular store that later became another one of my supporters. She was a little shorter than me, and had a round face that was so jolly that you couldn't help but smile when she spoke to her. I asked her for some help to figure out what size I was, and she was surprised I didn't know.

"How is it possible you don't know your size, girl? You have been living in a cave or something?"

Her comment made me chuckle, and I gave her a simple explanation that I had just had gastric band surgery. She was intrigued that she had found someone who had the surgery, and asked many questions on the process. I answered them while she went to grab a tape measure, and another woman standing by joined our conversation. Both ladies said they had considered weight loss surgery, but were afraid of what could happen. I told them I understood, but told them the benefits I had experienced in the last two months.

My jovial assistant said she would start measuring to see my bra size. She explained the process, and I shook my head to show I understood what she was about to do. She stretched the measuring tape around my body, and then paused.

"Girl, first of all, you need to get some new bras. I can tell you right now that the one you are wearing right now is too big."

I do need to share that I have always been a heavy chested girl, which is the one set of assets that boys have never seemed to mind complimenting me on. Before surgery, I had grown to be a 48 DDD, which I know draws some gasp from people. Honestly, I never had a problem with The Pointer Sisters (Yes, I named my chest) being so large, but there are negatives. It kills your back, and with all the problems I had, the sisters were killing my posture. I still loved them though, and I really never thought that the sisters would change dramatically.

I looked down at my chest and realized that it was a bit smaller, and the bra I was wearing was not giving The Pointer Sisters their best performance. I did need a bra, but what size was I?

After hoisting up my bra straps the assistant went around my body and did some measuring, and finally announce my bra size.

"Girl, you are a 46DD. It's time for a new bra."

To understand the significance of this size, you need to know that my bra size in high school was a 44DD. No joke, my chest was that size, I just made sure to wear a sports bra (sometimes two sports bras) to cover up the mounds. To hear my bra size was smaller than its measurements when I was 30 was astonishing! How had I lost that much fat in one area? I smiled and the associate asked my old bra size. When I shared it with her she clapped her hands like a child and said "Yay" to me. She deserves a raise for what she does, especially after she helped me find a new bra to take home.

She led me around the store, looking for cheap clothes to try on. I was a size 24 at this point, which was a big change since I was a 26/28 before surgery. I bought three shirts and said "thank you" multiple times to the associate before I left.

She smiled and handed me my bag, and exclaimed, "Good bye to the incredible shrinking woman!"

When I return to the store she still calls me this, and it cracks me up that she remembers me.

Another bra experience that I had was actually with a former student. Jasmine was such a joy to have in the classroom two years before my surgery. She was a plus size girl, and she was so beautiful, especially her face and smile. She was an associate at a plus size clothing store in the mall through her high school years, and she stayed there when she began attending college. I would go to visit her from time to time, and grab some cheap clothing while she strolled around the store with me, sharing the latest drama of her life.

Before the surgery, Jasmine had always told me I was pretty, and I would roll my eyes at her comments of wanting my hips. She was silly girl, but an entertaining one to have in my life day in and day out. I was so glad to go into the store and to see her to take on this new adventure of smaller clothing shopping.

She did her traditional grin when I entered the store, and gave me a big hug. She asked me how my health was, and how different I felt. I caught her up on everything, and she giggled at my odd new thinner me facts. I told her I was bra shopping, and she squealed with delight.

"Oh, Ms. Mathews! We are about to make those breast be poppin' with this new body!" was her battle cry before taking me into the lingerie department.

She went from rack to rack, picking up the styles she said that would look good on me. She found one with a dipping line so I could wear a shirt that was low cut, she found one that would make The Pointer Sisters look firmer, and she found a universal bra that I could use when I needed to go strapless. All I did was follow her, and answer an occasional question of what color I wanted in each style she chose. With each style she would grab and put in the air for me to see, I would simple say, "Black one please" and she would grab it. After going to each rack of her favorite styles, she took me to the dressing room.

While putting her key in the door, she said, "Do you have a problem with putting them on and showing me how they look? And don't act funny to that question because you were my teacher. This is my job woman, and if you are about to spend this money, I gotta make sure you're looking good. So don't give me a funny look."

The question did startle me because I hadn't "posed" in clothing for anyone in a long time. There was no way I was modeling a bra for someone before surgery. If someone wanted to see a rack of rolls, they needed to go to the bakery, and not watch me half nude. The idea of showing off my bras to someone was weird, and the fact it was a former student added another layer of bizarreness to the partial nudity.

But Jas was right, it was her job, and I would be offended if someone wouldn't let me do what I knew best. I couldn't say "No" to showing her because she was the associate, and I was about to drop a decent amount of money on some new bras.

So, I did as instructed. I put them on, open the fitting room door, and posed in each bra that she chose. Before showing Jas, I would look myself over, and I marveled that for the first time in a long time, I had a waist. And suddenly I realize I had an extremely defined hour glass figure. Where did this come from?

There was an emotional event with each bra I put on, seeing my new figure in different styles, and examined my own new personal shapes. Jasmine approved most of her choices each time I opened the door.

I had to have her stare, and spin around, and have her make sure the bra straps were adjusted correctly. She was right, she did know what she was doing, and she was right on her choices to make my body look more balanced. We both agreed on the best two choices, the neck plunging bra and the one I could use when wearing strapless shirts and dress. They made my body look fantastic, and Jasmine liked them so much she clapped.

After I changed back into my clothes, and came out the room to purchase my bras, Jasmine told me to keep up the good work. Lastly, she stated, "And now I definitely want those hips, Ms. Mathews."

I stopped at a couple more stores and picked up a couple things. I bought jeans from a store I hadn't been able to shop in for years due to my size. I bought some t-shirts at a local store and found out that I had to give up my 3XL size for a 2XL, and even then that size was loose on me. I didn't know how to react, and I realized what people meant to becoming a shopaholic. I loved buying new clothes! It was fun, and exciting, and an important part of my transformation. I was becoming something new, and I liked it.

THE EMOTIONAL, THE HORMONAL, AND THE ACNE

To write just about the positives of having gastric banding surgery would be keeping the idea of weight loss in a fantasy land. The truth is, there are negative issues with the surgery too. I went quite a while until I started to experience the tirade of annoyance known as the emotional, the hormonal, and the acne.

You need to know that before the surgery, I was not an emotional person. I was not the one to cry through movies, or to show emotions for others to see. I hate crying, with a passion, and I try to keep my tears hidden behind closed doors. I once remember watching a movie with friends and all my girlfriends were crying, except me. Of course I thought the love story was sad. I felt some emotions toward the heroine, who was supposed to lose her love, and I felt a knot in my throat, but tears just did not come. One of my friends said I was callus, which wasn't true. I felt emotion, but I just didn't like to display it around people. I am the tough one, and I always have been. That was easy for me before I had the surgery. Afterward was another story.

I often cried in the years after surgery. I still do my crying behind closed doors, but there would be days that I would be so stressed that I had to cry to feel better. Being patient for change is a draining aspect of having the gastric banding, and making so many changes in one's life all at once can make one overly emotional. I would cry when I was happy, and I would cry when I was frustrated. I cried when I went under 300, and I cried when I put on my biggest pair of pants, and they didn't fit anymore. I cried in fitting rooms when I caught a glimpse of my new body in a window walking to class, and when I realized, I could jog again. I was a hot mess of emotions, and there was nothing I could do about it. It felt good to cry sometimes. It was such a new experience for me to be overwhelmed with joy. I could have been a spokesperson for a tissue brand.

One side effect that I didn't enjoy was my changes in hormones. My "lady issues" began in junior high, and I have struggled with them ever since. From menstrual cycles that had no pattern, to birth control pills, to cyst, to tumors, to polyps, to Endometriosis, I had all the problems a woman could have except cancer. It is a major part of my weight gain, and I had hoped that these issues would be behind me. One of the positives that lead me to having the surgery was the possibility of ending my issues with PCOS, which is Poly Cystic Ovarian Syndrome. To give you a health lesson, everyone woman has cysts on their ovaries at least once a month, so that is not the problem. It becomes a serious problem when you are a woman like me, who can have multiple cysts on your ovary at one time. The largest number found in one of my ultrasounds was five on one ovary, and it was beyond painful. PCOS can happen when the body produces too much insulin, and in having the surgery, my insulin level would decrease, which meant fewer cysts in my body.

I celebrated the idea of ending my "lady issues" and counted the days for my issues to disappear. Well, I am still counting.

Granted, since surgery I haven't had a cyst or a tumor. I did celebrate that day after having an ultrasound come back with the all clear (and yes; I cried over this too), but I am still suffering in different areas.

Once you have this surgery, your hormones can have mixed messages on what is going on. It's like your body going into shock from all the change, and its first action is to react. My endocrine system fought me like Ali fought Fraizer and made sure to let me know that I would be taking some body shots for making such a drastic change to my way of life.

My menstrual cycle decided to make an appearance whenever it felt like it. It came so infrequently that Bill and I used code words for my lady issues. I understand that using the classic term of "Aunt Flo" is not politically correct to some, but it made it easier to keep track of my unwanted visitor. Sometimes Aunt Flo would arrive on time, sometimes she decided to stay over for an extended amount of time, and sometimes she would leave and come right back a week later.

I hated Aunt Flo with every fiber of my being, and she let me know that she was unhappy with my new lifestyle. She would keep me in bed on the weekends because I would have no energy, or I would be hurting from her punches. She made me grouchier than usual, which lead to me wanting isolation from others, and she cost me extra money because she needed the right accommodations and medications. She was one of the worst parts of having to deal with the changes of my body, and, due to having a blood clot years earlier; I couldn't take anything to control her. Also, my body chemistry was altered by my hormones, which meant I sweated all the time. I would have to change my clothes two times a day, and shower constantly. Nothing could help me with the sweating, and I couldn't stand the feel of moisture all over my body. I sometimes woke up in the middle of the night drenched in sweat, and then the next night the opposite would happen, I would have extreme chills. My hormones were not happy, and neither was I.

My family doctor felt bad for me and told me to make my heating pad my best friend during these times. He explained that some gastric banded patients struggle with their hormones for years, and until my body settled into the new me, I would have to toughen up and deal with her wrath. I was miserable with all these issues, but the worst had not appeared yet, the acne.

I have never had a major issue with acne, not even when I was a teenager. Granted, I remember grabbing a medicated pad once in a while, but nothing so major that my whole face suffered an acne invasion. That changed after surgery, and my face that had always had beautiful, clear skin became covered with acne.

It started small on my forehead, and overnight my acne went from three small bumps to my entire forehead having craters like the moon. It didn't stop there; my new issue invaded my chin. Each bump was inflamed and tremendously sore to the touch, and it continued to grow in number. I washed my face with soap, with acne scrub, with name brand products that promised relief, and nothing helped the issue. I ordered expensive skin care products from home shopping parties. I had slathered my face before I went to bed, again when I woke to start my day, and a third time when I returned home after work. Nothing helped. Acne had started to control my life, and I now understood why teenagers freaked at their appearance in my classroom over zits.

I tried to cover up my issues with make-up, but it didn't work. To make matters worse, when the acne did come to a head and pop, it left a terrible dark scar on my skin or a sore, and my face became disgusting to me. I searched websites to see what I could do about this issue without spending more money, but I didn't find too many answers. Everyone just kept saying that time will help it, and it would just go away. A week after week, I grew more and more fearful of looking in the mirror at my face because the acne just kept coming.

One night, after discovering a new colony of zits, I went to my best friend with a face filled with sorrow and covered with acne medication. He knew how unhappy I had become with all the side effects from the surgery. I had started to become depressed dealing with my sweating, my bumpy face, and the need for the strongest of medication on the market to deal with my cramps. He said to me, "Would you rather be heavy again and have pretty skin and no visitations from Aunt Flo?"

No, I would never want to be heavy again. Despite these major annoyances, I know I can't go back to the old me. I just wished the new me wasn't so complicated.

There is hope. Some of my issues were a passing phase, but some are still going on now. I finally found the right combination medication for my skin and my acne went away, and the sweating issue only happens every once and awhile. My lady issues continue, but I can't have everything go away.

There are other minor side effects I have from time to time: nausea, heartburn, bruising, and other annoying issues, but nothing that can stop be from enjoying my new health and body. The best thing is to be patient and keep working on improving yourself, and everything will hopefully fall into place.

BACK TO WORK

The last days of summer passed, and suddenly I was faced with the reality of returning to school. Summer school is much easier than doing a regular school day, and the idea of getting back into the daily grind of the education world saddened me. I didn't know how people would react to me, and I didn't know if I was ready to answer all the questions and hear about all the rumors that would circle about me.

I am sure that my workplace is not any different than most people in the workforce. There are the supportive people, the complainers, the gossips, the free spirits, the positive energy people, and, of course, the haters. My first days included all these groups.

Teachers are required to go back to school about a week before the kids do. To be honest, most teachers go in before the required time to get a grip of their classrooms and to get things in order with lesson plans. It angers me when people make such silly comments of teachers have so much time off. To be truthful, if teachers didn't have time off, they would probably become emotionally and mentally unstable. I did go back a couple days before my required date, and worked silently in my room where no one would find me behind the closed door, and slipped out unnoticed. But I would be noticed on the first official day, and I had to brace myself for the groups at my workplace.

First of all, the majority of people in my workplace are amazing people. CA is a community that knows how to be supportive at the right time and involved in all kinds of community service and kind acts. It's not a phony act that most people put on for the public;

it's just that most people of CA know how to be a real community member.

I walked in for the first day of school meetings, and people from all the groups greeted me and had questions. Some members of the gossipers asked me about the weight loss so that they could tell the others. Positive people came by personally when I was working to share cheers and hugs. In general, the first day back was pretty easy to deal with, but that was because the haters were waiting in the wings for the next couple days.

Those who choose to join the banded club (I call them bandits) need always to keep in mind the following phrase, "Haters are gonna hate." It doesn't matter what you say or what you do, those people who are haters will never be on your side. Their main goal is to make sure to make you feel crappy, and to second guess every decision you make. Haters will try to get you to cheat on your diet. Haters will talk about you behind your back and smile in your face, and haters will come and ask you some of the most annoying questions just to get under your skin. My best advice, put a hater in their place and then move along, because, like I stated earlier, haters are going to hate, no matter what.

My main encounter with a hater happened on the third day back. I was walking to my classroom when a coworker stopped me. She started pleasant enough, and we discuss the summer casually before she questioned my loss of weight. She had heard I had surgery from the gossips, but she felt that she needed to ask that key question that would take away any feelings of success.

"Do you feel guilty that you are cheating to lose weight?"

So now I am cheating. I guessed when life did what it did to me it was fair. I guess that when I started to gain weight from medication in college that was fair. That I had a fear to eat in front of people in restaurants at one point due to the label the fat girls eat everything is fair. That my blood clot medicine that made me become the heaviest was "fair." I wanted to smack my lips at her say, "Girl, bye."

I didn't give a damn about the fair in losing my weight. I didn't need to explain anything to this person, but due to my smart mouth when challenged, I gave a reply.

"Life hasn't been fair to me, so I used its game against it. I guess I won this time."

The person said that I looked great and then walked away quickly down the hall. As I said, haters are going to hate.

It was a different story with my students. Kids don't have a filter, especially teenagers. My students say whatever they feel needs to be said, and sometimes this is a good thing, and sometimes it could crush a weak individual. One thing you know you will receive from teenagers is brutal honesty.

There were students overjoyed with the change. They came to the room, and said such kind words and gave such loving hugs for my new success. I had kids whispering about me in the hall, and tattle tales to come back and tell me what was said. I chuckled at some of the brutal comments, and my personal favorite from a kid who said I was looking "damn fine" the first week of school.

There were some children who didn't approve.

I have amazing relationships with some of my students. I have kids who keep contact with me and become friends as they reach adulthood. I had two students who frowned at the changes that I was very close to, James and Shariel.

Now, they didn't think me the losing weight was necessarily a bad thing, they just thought it was different.

I had taught James and his older brother, Edgar, in my tenure at CA. James and I had become close during his freshman year, and we continued to talk up to this day. He came to see me and looked at me strangely, and I could tell that he disapproved of something. I asked him what was wrong.

"I just feel that you are not Ms. Mathews anymore."

His statement stung. I questioned him on why he would say that.

"My Ms. Mathews was just motherly looking I guess. I didn't see her as heavy or skinny, I just saw her as a mom. Right now, you don't look like a mom anymore. I still love you, but it's just different."

I had never thought my appearance would change students views of me. I guess I was just wrapped up with losing the weight for me and not thinking how it would affect those kids in my classroom that looked up to me. To be honest, I cared more about what the kids thought than the people I worked it.

I assured James that I was the same person and that I hoped he would be able to accept the non-matron looking version of Ms. Mathews compared to the "Momma" Mathews that he was used to. He giggled and said he would give the new me a chance.

Shariel had a problem with how quickly the weight had come off. She stated that she thought I would be 20 pounds thinner when we came back, but I was closer to 30, and it freaked her out.

"You don't have to lose it all in one month, woman! Slow down! Soon, I won't be able to see you."

Shariel had a point, the weight was coming off so quickly in the beginning, and it was something for everyone to get used to, especially me. My promise was that I would not starve myself and that she could yell at me if I dropped another 30 by the time she graduated in June. She agreed.

I did feel different the first semester of returning to school.

I walked around my work place easier. I didn't get tired, and I didn't get out of breath like I use to. I found myself almost never sitting behind my desk during the school day. My work clothes style changed, and I became flashy. Everything with my work self-changed, my looks, my attitude, and most importantly, my energy level.

I had more energy at the end of the day, and I didn't want to collapse when the bell rang (well, not most days). And there were two key areas where things improved: my back and my feet.

The main areas of change were two areas that I never thought would get better. The weight on my feet from standing would make me want to scream at the end of the day. As the old phrase goes, my dogs would be barking. I would get home, and they would pulsate with pain. And my back was always a mess. Now granted, I still have back problems, but not at the level that I did before the surgery. By the end of the school year, the old me would be planted behind that desk because my body couldn't take it, but the new body had adapted well to the work environment. So in many ways, I think the weight loss made me a better teacher.

So, I let the supports stay in my corner. I listened to those who cared, and I left the haters and gossipers behind in my workday. Things settled down and became normal once.

FAT FLASHBACK-I BREAK THINGS...

Everyone breaks things. Children handle objects that are supposed to be forbidden and lose their grip, those who grow older blame destructive behavior of breakage on their weakening eyes, and some people are filled with clumsiness. I use to break things, but I broke things for another reason. I broke things because I was too fat.

We have all seen the comical happening of a fat person sitting on some item and the slow snapping of the object, and then, the sudden crumble to the floor. It is hilarious...unless you are the breaker. I have been the breaker in some amazing comedy routines, sometimes in private, and sometimes for the world to see.

There is nothing more terrifying to a fat person than the idea of breaking something in front of people. It's even scary to break things in front of your family.

The main thing I use always to break was my bed. Growing up, I had to share a bedroom with sister. My sister and I had bunk beds, and during our elementary days, they were stacked. I slept on the top bunk for a while, but with my growing weight problems there had to be a fear of me crashing through the mattress and smashing Angi, so we decided to debunk the beds.

My father worked for General Motors, which was decent money, but not great money. For me to think that my father would be able to run out and buy me a new bed would be me being foolish. Each time I broke my bed, he had to use some handyman skills, which, despite my love for my father, I have to admit were quite limited.

I remember waking one morning and hearing a slight pop at the foot of the bed. My first thought was to freeze my body and to be as stiff as a mummy. I even went so far as to holding my breath, which I don't know why that seems to be the fat person method for the inevitable snapping of the furniture. I next tried to slide my way off the bed, but it didn't help. Half of the bed popped, and I toppled toward the end of my bed.

I didn't want to tell my parents. I was so embarrassed and so scared that I would get yelled at. I didn't get in trouble for breaking my bed, but the family did joke about my big booty doing the damage. It was alright, I would have teased too, but it was a stinging reminder that I was large, and my weight was destructive.

I broke my bed about four times over the years, and dad always fixed it. I remember him going out and buying these huge silver bolts to put it back together the last time. I knew that if I broke it after this time of heavy pounds, there were no bolts that could fix the mess, and I would be sleeping on the floor.

But breaking my bed wasn't the worst item I broke. The worst happened in my late 20s, in front of over 40 men.

As I stated earlier, I use to own a semi-professional football team, where I was "Boss Lady". We were having a football combine, which was a tryout for players for the season. Former players came and gave greetings to me, and newer players looked at me amazed because I was a chick who would soon possibly own their football careers. After doing greetings and public relations activities, I grabbed a folding chair to sit down and talk to one of my favorite (and most attractive) players, Eric, better known as "Hollywood."

While "Hollywood" and I were talking, I felt a sliding sensation with my chair but paid it no mind because I believed it was the turf underneath me making it sinks a bit. It wasn't the turf. It was my weight and it popped the screws of the folding chair. When I realized what was happening, it was too late for me to hop out the chair.

There was a quick snap. Then a total collapse. Then me laying on the turf. I had broken the chair in front of everyone.

I was sprawled out on top of the broken chair, and I couldn't get up. Eric ran to pick me up, along with four other guys. My hand got caught in the broken legs of the chair. After people scrambling to pick me up and digging out my fingers in the parts of the chair, I was back up on my feet, and wanting to run to my car.

Everyone was concerned that I was fine, but I know that people had a great laugh at my fat girl spill when they weren't around me. The cherry on top of the fat girl fall was I fractured my finger and had to put ice on it for the rest of the event. As I said, I break things.

My fatness made me break things, and made me destroy clothes. I split some pants over the years, and even more notoriously, I have rubbed inner thighs out of many pairs of sweats and jeans.

I once rubbed a hole in my favorite sweatpants in fifth grade, and there was a huge hole that you could see if you walked behind me. I had no idea until a kid made fun of me walking home from the bus stop. My thighs had embarrassed me again.

You would think that a fat girl would get used to these mishaps, but it never got easier. My hopes were to get to a point where I could sit in tiny chairs with ease, and run and flop on my bed without having flashbacks after having the surgery.

FITNESS

As my size changed, so did my need for fitness. Now, a normal person would want to ease into a slower level of fitness, but not this woman. Oh no, I wanted to do something adventurous, something I would never have done at my larger size. I decided that I would take pole dancing classes.

I do have to begin by saying that I now have a new respect for girls who make their living by twirling on a pole for patrons for one dollar bills. I had no idea how many muscle groups that a person uses when performing this activity, but I learned that very quickly when I started my new fitness classes.

My fascination with performing this fitness started from attending a bachelorette party for my friend, Heidi. This party had some of the wildest women in Flint in attendance, and it consisted of an instructor teaching basic moves and lots of alcohol. Watching these women of multiple sizes trying to work that pole was hilarious, but it also did build a level of sexiness for each woman in attendance. I didn't do too bad in the party lesson, and I won the label of being the most flexible on that pole. The instructor said we could come back for lessons, and many talked about it but didn't sign up. I took the chance and decided to take more classes.

For my first day of "pole" school, I put on some sweats and a comfortable t-shirt and arrived five minutes early. There were stretching exercises, and words of why this was now an acceptable way of providing fitness for the "every day" woman. I listened to every word and was excited to learn how to perform on the pole.

The first day was pretty much like the lesson I had at the bachelorette party, with a new couple moves. I concentrated on learning everything and made it through the first part of the routine with no issues. I went home excited, and eager to learn the next moves to strengthen my body. That was the last time I was excited about the class.

I went for more lessons and learned more moves, but I suddenly became very uncomfortable. My second lesson went fine, and I was getting better at working around that pole, but the third was the start of my downfall in pole fitness.

The instructor commented on my clothing. I was wearing sweat or long shirt to class, and I needed to dress so my skin could grip the bar. For me to continue to learn the next stages, I would need to wear booty shorts or boy-cut underwear.

I wasn't ready for that, not even in front of women. Everyone else in the class was fit, and skinny, and tall. I was the opposite of all those girls. I did concede and wear shorts and rolled them up some, but that didn't work. I couldn't grip the bar, and I soon learned I couldn't do the advanced level moves because my arms couldn't hold up my weight.

I felt like the fat kid in gym class, that the teacher gave pep talks to try and make them feel like they were improving, but everyone knew that I was going nowhere. I couldn't do the advanced moves, and my self-esteem was right back to when I was 318 pounds.

One time I tried to hold my weight up and I hit the floor, hard. My back thumped from the pain, and my hands burned from slipping off the bar. I walked out of that class so sad, and I didn't go back. I was heartbroken because I wanted to be fit again and to do something that made me feel sexy, but I felt the opposite when I left that class.

I was sad for a couple weeks after failing at my pole adventures, but I decided to try a new form of fitness soon after that, roller skating.

You need to know that I hadn't been skating since middle school and did to some crazy ideas of my co-workers, I considered joining roller derby. I thought it sounded like a cool idea, and I even went to see some bouts to see how the sport worked.

Being the perfectionist that I am, I refused to try-out for the sport without getting the basics of skating down. I didn't think that I could balance, let alone knock someone down in a competitive sport like roller derby.

I decided to pay for skating lessons. I made arrangements with the local skating rink to come in for lessons on Saturday mornings before the skating opened for the younger patrons. I felt a tad foolish signing up for skating lessons at my age, but, if I truly wanted to give this roller derby thing a try. I would need to know the basics and get my skating legs back under me.

I arrived five minutes early for my lessons to a cold and dark rink. There were a few lights on, and there was a figure skating class happening when I walked through the doors. The four girls skating looked adorable and were decked out in pretty pink, blue, and white sequined outfits with lots of ruffles. I stopped and admired their skating abilities, and realized that they couldn't be over the age of 10. A wave of terror came over me.

Who would be in the class with me?

Would I fall and hurt myself?

Would people laugh at me?

The answers to these questions were answered in of two hours.

I wanted help to get my rental skates and noticed a small boy with his grandfather. Dear Jesus, I was about to skate with a small boy? Here I am, a 30+-year-old woman taking lessons with a small boy! It couldn't get any worse than this!

Oh, but it did.

While putting on my roller skates, an older woman with a five-year-old girl walks in. The little girl has on a precious pink coat, and her hood up covering her face. The older woman, talks to a person up front, and is directed to the same spot I picked up my skates. I was taking skating lessons with a young boy and a five-year-old little girl.

To make matters even more interesting, the instructor was a sub for the "real" instructor. She was a nice woman, and she told me I was very brave to put skates back on for lessons. She asked me what level of experience I had with skating as an adult. My reply made her giggle.

"My level is about a negative 7. I want to get to level zero so I can be proud of myself."

I was told to skate out to the center. With every ounce of my concentration, I made it safely. I did have one major problem; I couldn't remember how to stop. I think I only stopped because I ran out of momentum. My instructor smiled and said she would make sure I knew how to stop correctly before I left that day.

She did teach me how to stop. She also taught me how to get correctly up when I fell, which I am proud to say I didn't do the first day. I was trained how to skate with my hands out of my hoodie sweatshirt, how to look up instead of staring at the floor in fear, and how to march in my skates.

My skating counterparts had lessons of their own. My young man, who was nine, did many of the lessons with me. He was a determined boy, and sometimes skated too fast for his skill level and fell many times. To his credit, he popped right back up like a heavyweight boxer, no matter how many times he hit that pavement. The little girl was more of a hassle than a learner. I know that a person should keep in mind that she was a five-year-old, but she also was a child that did not want to be there. She crawled all over the floor, wouldn't listen to directions, and insisted that she needed to go play the arcade games instead of learning how to skate. It wouldn't have annoyed me so much if the older lady (who turned out to be a grandma) would have come and gotten her, but she did no such thing. As a matter of fact, I don't even think that granny was paying attention, because she sat and read her newspaper the entire time and gave no assistance to the instructor.

The cherry on top of my embarrassment sundae was the rink letting in people before opening hours. A large party of adults and children walked in to see me taking skating lessons with two young children. I wanted to hide from embarrassment, and as soon as the lesson was finished I pulled on the wall to the nearest bench to hurry and take my skates off and run out the rink.

While I was trying to finish unlacing my second skate, the little girl's grandmother came by and stopped in front of me. I stopped and looked up at her, halfway expecting her to curse at me for frowning at her grand baby for getting in the way of me skating twice during the lesson.

"Girl, I give you credit. It takes some nerve to learn how to skate as an adult. I don't have the strength that you do. Do yo' thang girl, do yo' thang."

We both giggled, and I thanked her. She never came back, and neither did her granddaughter, but my young male skater came for one of the next lessons. I finished my skating lessons and stayed afterward for open skate to practice what I learned. I stumbled, fell, sweated, and I got better. It was one of the best fitness classes that I took, and it turns out it is an easy way to burn calories. It was a wonderful way for me to stay focused on losing the weight, and both my instructors were great.

Unfortunately, the plan for roller derby fell apart, so I didn't continue skating, but I think about my skates often. One day I will pick them back up.

I did other fitness classes after that: Sexy Flexi workouts, yoga, and then my favorite, belly dancing. Bellydi was my favorite, and the instructor, Azziza, was so full of energy. It was a nonstop workout, and she waited for no one. I took this class for months, and then I started doing home workouts for belly dancing. My midsection was getting smaller, and most importantly, it was starting to get a little toned. My hour glass shape was starting to come into place, and I loved it.

You can't get banded and expect for it to do all the work for you. A banded person needs to have some fitness outlet. It doesn't have to be as odd as my choices, but you need to see that you can do different things because you are different when you lose the weight. It takes time to find what is best for you, but I found some great options. One day, I hope to spin on that pole again and to knock someone off their skates, but until that day, I will keep searching for the fitness fix.

FAB FLASHBACK-GETTING PEOPLE'S ATTENTION

I was once told by another banded person that I would get sick of hearing people say that I was "thinner" or "skinny". She said that she became annoyed with those words and the phrases referring to the change. I haven't gotten to that point yet in my new life, but I do have a different problem. I am clueless on people seeing me differently and giving me not only verbal compliments, but nonverbal clues. Other people notice for me, but I never notice them when it is first brought to my attention. It's pretty sad because time has passed, and I still don't get why people give me so much attention.

The first big attention moment happened at a bowl game the day after Christmas. As I mentioned earlier, Bill is a broadcaster, and he and my father teamed together to create the Michigan Regional Sports Network, an Internet broadcasting company. One of the cool perks of hanging out with the boys is attending sporting events and living the good life with press credentials. We have done this a couple times, but the excitement of free food, press passes to the field and hanging out with big wigs in the press never gets old to me.

The best perk of being part of the press is being able to walk down on the field and being with the teams in the final minutes of the battle between the trenches. I love that moment of walking down the tunnel (the same tunnel that professional football players walk down each Sunday), and entering a field to see thousands of spectators in the stands. It's breathtaking, and before surgery is was extremely breathtaking to haul all that weight down that tunnel and to realize I had sweat running down my face from the trip. This time down the tunnel, I didn't have the sweat, I didn't have to gasp for air, and I didn't have my feet pulsating because of the pressure walking down the hill.

I don't know if I was enjoying my fit moment, enjoying looking into the stands, or enjoying the play on the field that prevented me from finding out that I had personal fans. Bill had already noticed and walked up behind me with a toothy grin.

"Aren't you going to acknowledge your fans?"

I turned to him and frowned.

"What are you talking about now, William?"

"I knew you didn't notice your fan club; maybe you should turn around and look at them"," was Bill's reply.

I dipped my chin down into my chest and then turned my head slightly to the right to peer over my shoulder. There was a group of five guys, probably college recruits, standing 20 yards behind me. It looked to me like they were watching the game, and I shared that information with Bill. He was still convinced that I had a fan club.

We argued quietly about his observations for awhile, and then Bill offered up a clever proposal.

"OK, I want you walk down the field 15 yards and then just stand there. If those boys follow, we both know that I am right."

I agreed, and after the referee had called a time-out on the field, I moved down 15 yards and stood next to the camera man. I waited a couple minutes and then turned around.

The boys had followed me. Bill was right, and I was wrong. I stared for a moment at the group, which lead to one of them to smile and another one to wave.

Due to my lack of experience with receiving the attention I just smiled back and turned back to the game. Bill came a moment later, giggled, and said, "I told you so."

I received attention at school. Teenage boys began to express inappropriately that I was their "dream woman" and in four years would come back to marry me. I reacted like any other teacher would. I told them to shut up.

I received flowers on Valentine's Day. On my birthday, cards would appear in my mailbox. Verbal invitations from students to "hook me up" with their older family members began to appear, and fathers looked at me differently at parent-teacher conferences. It was crazy to a girl like me to receive such attention, and I am still not use to it. I enjoy it, but I'm still not use to it.

I had moments like this with strangers in stores too.

While doing one of my compulsive shopping sprees at one of my favorite stores I had an unforgettable moment.

While looking over jeans, the manager of the store came to speak to me. She was a polite lady, who always greeted me when I came into the store.

"Excuse me, but you're so pretty. Have you thought about doing one of our fashion shows?"

My first reaction was simple. I laughed, loudly. I knew she couldn't be talking to me about modeling. But she was serious, and she began her promo about the store's upcoming event to premiere the winter line of the company and the need for models for the event. I told her I didn't know about doing any modeling and was sure that she could find someone else that was more qualified to strut on the catwalk in their new clothes. The manager was very animated that I should join in the festivities, and oddly, a woman in the store joined in and told me that she thought I could be a great model for the event. After much persuasion, I gave permission for the manager to call in a couple days, and I would give her an answer.

I went home and thought about it. Me? A model? It just seemed so ridiculous. The idea of me strutting around showing off clothes seems so preposterous. Who would want to see me as a model?

I would.

I would like to see me as a model. And that's why I went back into the store a day later and spoke to the same manager, and said I would participate.

The first interesting aspect in modeling is doing a "fitting". The whole point of doing a fitting is to find an outfit that flatters you and entices the attendees to want to buy the outfit on the spot. You have to have a complete outfit, which means you needed to even have accessories that make the buyer want to spend more at the store. My outfit was to be an everyday ensemble, which anyone would want to wear. It was a beige, bell collar sweater, a pair of dark blue, boot cut jeans. My wintertime accessories were a tan, plaid scarf, gold earrings, tan boots filled with soft foam, and a plaid hat.

I liked my outfit and thought it made me look nice for the event. After the fitting, I received instructions on the day and was asked to tell everyone to come for the big event. I posted my new adventure on social networks, and people cheered my efforts of trying out modeling.

When the day arrived, I felt like a diva. I was given a make-up session and learned some new tricks to putting on makeup and making my skin look clearer. I was then rushed to change into my outfit. It looked as fabulous as the first day I tried it on. Before the actual fashion show started, I was used as a living mannequin in the store to show off my fancy duds. People came up to me to look at the outfit and to compliment how nice it looked on me. I wondered if I would have done this before losing the weight, and the answer was simple, "no". I would never have let people walk up and compliment me on my looks, and I wouldn't have been confident enough to model clothes. The biggest event was the catwalk. Simply put, it was my job to sell the clothes to the attendees, which meant they wanted me to walk with confidence in front of everyone while they described my garments. I had to wait until it was my turn. When announced, I walked through the crowd with my head held high to show off my attire. Cameras flashed, people clapped, and I felt like a star. Afterward, people told me what a great job I did, and how beautiful I was, and for once, I believed in the comments of strangers.

I left the event with some new clothes and a better attitude about my looks. I was still in amazement that a woman could walk up to me and say I was pretty, and for random strangers to agree. I continue to do the fashion shows as a diva model to this day and always enjoy the feeling of being a showgirl in fashion. The Battle with the "O-Beast."

As time passed, I realized that I had easily fallen in and out of love with many things. This is a typical process for any "GB" member I would suspect. You realize you're feeling about some of these items and events. You have a secret celebration or mourning period within your soul.

There were many things that I had fallen in love with that I stated earlier: fitness, flirting, and shopping, but I developed other odd "loves" that most people would not understand.

I developed a love for different foods that I couldn't stand before. My palette had changed tremendously in this quest for health, and I started eating things that I turned my nose up at in the past or didn't dare eat before.

Many of the foods I ate during my healing stages after surgery didn't stay on my regular menu, but some of them became delicious options on my plate.

I never gave up re-fried beans; it was a must if I went to have Mexican food. I became excited if I found someone who could make outstanding re-fried beans, which was food I would usually choose to not have on the menu.

There were others: catfish, beets, feta and goat cheese, grape leaves with rice and meat, bruschetta, sugar-free fruit drinks, pickles, and pita chips with any dip. It was insane to see my new food choices! I would never have made these choices before the surgery, but these were good foods for me to have, and they were delicious.

I have always loved to read, but I developed a love of reading food labels. I realized that you need to know what you are putting into your body, and how much a "true" serving was of many items. So many things are labeled healthy for you in the market, but they can be high is sodium, or the portion inside would be different than what the average person would eat in one sitting. I developed a love for being informed about my food intake and felt that I couldn't be lazy in knowing my food's contents.

I fell in love with simple things. I loved that I could get onto a massage table and not worry that it would snap. I loved that I could go to staff meetings in the auditorium, and I wouldn't have to sit on the edge of the tiny chairs. I loved that I could sometimes buy a smaller shoe because my feet didn't swell as much from working all day. I loved that I could try on rings in regular stores, and I loved to wear a belt. Those things are events that the common person wouldn't think twice about, but when you have battled with weight, you know that those are major joys in a person's life.

I have fallen out of love with many things, with the majority dealing with food.

I don't love all-you-can-eat places anymore. As a matter of fact, I despise them.

Oddly, during my first parts of college I worked at an all-you-can-eat place, and that was the time when I gained a lot of weight. I worked most nights smelling food being cooked on a grill or I would hear the popping of the bubbles in the deep fryer. At the end of the evening (depending on the manager) we were allowed to eat the leftover fried chicken, and my workplace made amazing fried wings. I would stuff my face, and during breaks I would waste my pile of ones from tips and would stay there and eat all I wanted at a discounted price. I use to love going to buffet-style places to eat. Now, they leave a bitter taste in my mouth.

I know that most people would say, "Well, just don't go to them." It is not that simple when you are part of my family.

Big celebrations have to be at an all-you-can-eat establishment. My family is quite large and quite diverse, and the thought is always to go somewhere where everyone can eat, laugh, sing celebratory songs, and then eat dessert.

I can't ask for family traditions to change because I did, so I have to fight through and attend. Just walking into those places makes my head and heart hurt. All the different food choices, all the fried items, all the dessert bars that can take care of any person's sweet tooth are overwhelming. Going to these places are painful for banded people like me because it is the Garden of Eden, or better yet, the Garden of "Eating".

The last visit was especially painful. It was my Grandma Edna's birthday, and everyone was meeting for the free for all attack on the items on the buffet. I walked in and the sight of all that food made me uneasy. But we always go here for Grams' birthday, and she was turning a very young 83. It was was her day.

You have to walk by the entire bar to get to the back room for the larger parties. I had to walk by all the meatballs, the glazed ham, the beloved fried chicken, and rolls lathered with butter. I glared at the starchy side dishes and the ice cream machine that seemed to have a permanent hum during business hours. Walking passed all those foods made me feel like I was Sean Pean in *Dead Man Walking. M*y knees buckling from weakness and watering of my eyes. I tried my best to keep my eyes forward, and not to stare at all the food goodness that was there for people to stuff themselves for happiness.

Whenever I did visit the food bar, I made sure to go to certain foods, and not to walk around and examine the food. Anyone who has gone to an establishment like this knows that everyone there looks like a rancher herding cattle. Flocks of people wandering around the food areas, bumping into one another, and hoping to beat someone to the last piece of chicken happens at all-you-can-eat joints. I didn't trust myself to do food grazing anymore; I had to be a girl with blinders on when it came to my food choices. I got ham, a small side of rice pilaf, a small spoon of mashed potatoes, and cabbage. That's it because those foods would go down with no problem, and I wouldn't feel guilty eating them. No, I don't want the Mac n Cheese, which was beckoning me to come over and visit. No,

I wouldn't go examine the dessert bar to be tempted by the golden caramel that dripped ever so slowing from the serving spoon onto some vanilla ice cream. I would fight temptation.

Another reason that I hated these places is that I knew I couldn't pile food on my plate, because everyone would see me and judge me. I couldn't come back with two plates of food choices to sample from because I knew that one relative would question me on what I was doing. I wouldn't and couldn't take that chance. To make matters worse there is always a store bought cake for the family celebration, and you are expected to take the cake and enjoy it. This time was so hard for me, and I had to fight temptation more than usual. No one knows of my struggles in these places, and I never said anything about it until now.

I have fallen out of love with holidays, and, once again, it is due to the food consumption. I didn't notice it before, but Americans are obsessed with connecting food to as many holidays as possible. I use to love Thanksgiving, Christmas, and Halloween, but not anymore. Holidays are just days for me to mess up my diet, and then feel sad that I didn't stay strong because I was surrounded by food. And it's not just those big three eating holidays, there's the Fourth of July, Mother's and Father's Day, Labor & Memorial Day, and the list goes on and on. We Americans eat for any reason at all, and it can make a banded person like me feel uneasy with holidays.

My job for the holidays is to make some of the most starch-filled foods, but they are my area of expertise. I am the beholder of the correct recipes for spaghetti and potato salad, and the sweets of cake and brownies. When it's a holiday, I am required to make at least one of these calorie ridden items, and it breaks my heart to cook them. I use to have such joys in cooking these items. Mostly because I would have to sample the food while preparing it, but I can't do that anymore, or I am taking in calories by snacking, which is one of my weaknesses.

I keep making these items, but I do it while battling the inner obese devil (I prefer to call that evil foe the "O-Beast".) I fight the "O-Beast" in wanting to eat throughout the cooking process, and then eating again at the family holiday gathering. So, I would, with great pity, cook the food and resist eating throughout the process and serve it to my family.

Before each holiday, I would ask what menu we would have, so I could look up the calories of each dish. Eating for the holidays when you are banded takes lots of planning and calorie counting. If there was barbecue, I needed to know what meat would be served so I wouldn't have something that had the possibility of getting stuck in my stomach. With the side dishes, I had to do the balancing game with points. I couldn't have potato salad and spaghetti salad, and I needed to have the foods that gave me protein so that I was staying healthy. Holidays are a constant juggling act of calorie points, the size of portions and emotions. Lord, how I hate the stress of holidays.

Sometimes the "O-Beast" would win on major holidays, and I would feel so guilty afterward. Usually, I would fail when it came to sweets, especially if there were some of my favorite junk foods on the counter. Cheesecake, chocolate cake, or other items with heavy icing would sucker me in at times, and I would go home and sulk. All I could do is be ready to fight the battle again in the next holiday, and go exercise to work off some of the calories.

Dealing with your loves and despising the unloved are all just part of the process of being banded, and you just fight day after day to keep yourself on track.

FAT FLASHBACK-SWIMSUIT TERROR

I haven't worn a swimsuit in over 20 years. That's right; I haven't enjoyed the freedoms of a swimming pool, of a Jacuzzi, a beach, or a fresh water establishment in over two decades. It is linked, once again, to a traumatic fat girl experience that I hope to get over in the upcoming years.

My swimsuit terror happened during gym class in junior high. Everyone knows that junior high was filled with many issues; every child is worried about their looks during that age. I was no different, and, of course, my main area of worries was my body. I had developed the nickname "Hips" at this point from my girlfriends, because my hips were well developed, along with many other parts below the waist. My hips were big, my butt was wide, and my main area of terror, were my thighs. I think the best way to describe my thighs and my legs are turkey drumsticks. My thighs were, and still are, very big, and very meaty pieces of flesh. My calves were short and muscular. It was my least favorite area on my body as a teenage girl, and I still feel that way.

My thighs are so large that I had to buy jeans a size bigger so that they could fit. I had the same problem with my uniform bottoms, and would have to stretch everything so that my thighs would not be an embarrassment. I was afraid of people pointing and laughing at the size, dimples, and waves in my thighs with everything that I wore.

So, in my telling about the extreme fear I had with my thighs completely covered up, you can image my fear with them totally exposed. You can't hide them with a swimsuit, they are out for the entire world to see and to evaluated.

I had to put on the swimming suit at school for my gym credit. It was required for all students to do one marking period of swim class for my school credit. I dreaded the idea, not only because of the swimsuit, but because I never learned how to swim. The class wasn't designed for nonswimmers like me because you were supposed to do laps, dive, and tread water, all of which I could not, and would not, do.

When the day came, I was miserable in the locker room. To add a layer to the humiliation, every girl had to strip down to put on their swimsuits. Some girls had no shame and did so out in the open. I was not that brave, and I ran into a bathroom stall. I was shaking in that stall while sliding on that swimsuit, and I wrapped a towel around myself as I emerged into the pool area.

I was thinking of ways to get out of swimming. I could say I was sick, or maybe try it's the "time of the month", but those were only temporary excuses. I needed to be tough and just struggle through the first day and pray that most people would not notice my thunder thighs.

After putting on the suit, I wrapped my torso in a bright blue beach towel. With my heading hanging low, I walked out to the pool to meet with the other classmates and my teacher.

I stayed wrapped up in the towel while my teacher did a speech about safety and how you had to swim to pass the marking period. There was no way out of this situation. Failing a class was more shameful than my thighs in my book, and I had to get in that pool.

"Alright boys and girls, leave your towels here and hop in the pool to start class."

Leave my towel? But the shallow end was all the way on the other side, which means I would have to walk in front of everyone with my thighs being seen. I didn't want to follow her directions, but I didn't want to get into trouble either. It was time to make a choice: defy the teacher and receive a consequence, or maybe listen to insults and be the object of gossip for the school day.

Maybe if I hustle to the other end, no one will have time to examine my body issue. I mean, others had to be nervous about their bodies at this point, and I could escape embarrassment. I had built up enough confidence to do it at this point; I was taking off that towel and walking to the other end.

Taking off that towel was a huge mistake.

After less than ten steps, a boy noticed my thighs. And he wanted all the other boys in class to notice them too. The boy pointed, and then started the insults. He talked about how huge they were, how they could feed a small country, how they were shaped like something he could order from Mr. Sanders, and other clever, but painfully hurtful insults. It felt like forever for me to get to the other end of that pool, and it was even worse when he made a comment about the water rising with me entering the shallow end.

I didn't run, and I didn't fake sick. I took the comments and the others giggling and pointing along with my aggressor. I hung my head at the end of the class. I quickly grabbed my towel to wrap my body like a mummy and trotted away into the locker room to hide, once again, in the bathroom stall.

This went on for a week. The same routine, the same feeling of shame for me each swimming lesson. The only thing that saved me was it turned out I was allergic to the chlorine in pools, and I was taken out of the swimming class and excused from it for the rest of the year. But the damage was done. I officially had a fear of swimsuits.

I went over 20 years without putting on a swimsuit. While other put on suits and other skimpy outfits during the summer, I always wore pants, no matter what the weather. I didn't dare lie out on a beach or jump in cool beach waters of Michigan because I couldn't have people stare at my thighs like they did when I was in middle school.

I finally went and tried on some suits due to the nagging of my beloved friend, Vera. Looking at my thighs still makes me uncomfortable, and I just couldn't bring myself to strut around in a swimsuit.

I don't think any amount of weight loss will change that, which proves that no matter how much you lose, you will always have default feelings about some aspect of your body. I will never be able to let go of the vision of those thunder thighs.

THE BEGINNINGS OF FAILURE

The first year and a half of life after surgery went better than expected. I keep losing weight little by little, and I became healthier. Life was good. Really good, but good things had to come to an end. Failure is always looming when someone is doing better in their lives, and when it sunk its claws and teeth into me, it tore away at my emotional flesh and rocked my soul to the core.

The failure began with sugar. After resisting its temptation for so long, I found out that I missed it so much, and that I needed a fix. Oddly, things filled with sugar could go down pretty easy. My stomach suddenly decided it didn't like some foods and the pain that jetted in my midsection and the center of my back let me know that was the case. Cookies went down easy, and my new favorite dessert, ice cream, slid down my system with ease. Sugar was always there to tempt me. It was to become my emotional fix during hard times. If I gave in, I felt extremely guilty.

Failure truly began in October. This one of the hardest months for teachers, along with the first couple weeks of November. It is when most educators go through the "teacher slump" in my district, and suddenly you realize that your body is just plain tired. I can't speak for all school districts, but the one I work in starts school in September and we don't get a break until Thanksgiving. You start to feel the effects of burnout in October, because those who work in high schools have to do homecoming, open houses, report card pick-up, and other events that are required to be smashed into the beginning of the calendar.

Along with all these other issues, I had received some troubling news. My grandfather, "Paw Paw" Evon, was sick. Other than my father, Paw Paw was the strongest man I knew. He had his health struggles like others, but he always bounced back from anything and everything. He, too, was a football coach, along with some other things, including working in different charities and events in the church. The only time that I had seen that man come anywhere near to submissive was the first time I saw him pray on his own.

My grandfather fought religion for a long time, and then suddenly, he gave God some credit. On one of our visits, my grandmother had me sneak and peek into her bedroom. There he was, on his knees, head bowed, and his hands clasped. I had never seen my grandfather give in to anything, so I thought that God being all powerful must be true to bring this man to his knees.

Nothing could take out my grandfather but God. I learned in October the second thing that could take him down. I learned that he had cancer.

Paw Paw was diagnosed with Stage 4 Bladder Cancer on Halloween, one of my favorite holidays. I always loved Halloween because it was a time for children to be so happy. Kids smiled because people complimented them on their cool costumes, they grinned when the received candy, and it left such lasting memories for all my family members. Now, the clearest memory I have of Halloween was my grandfather receiving a death sentence.

I found out the news from my sister by text message. Everyone else was in Kalamazoo at the hospital and received the news there. I just kept looking at the text, like it was a cruel joke or some spam from a business wanting money. It was true, my grandfather was dying.

With a cloudy mind, I went into Bill's room. He was doing his evening ritual, chatting with people on his laptop and listening to his music. He stopped pecking on the keys, looked up and me, and took off his headphones.

"What's up?"

"My grandfather is going to die. Soon."

"What are you talking about?"

I slowly handed him the phone, and he read the text.

"Jes, there are things that can be done, I'm sure the doctors will do their best…"

"Don't bullshit this, Bill! He's gonna die. My grandfather is gonna die, and it can't be fixed! I'm not ready for this. I just not ready. I'm…I'm"

I snatched the phone from out of his hand and stormed out. I went to my room, closed the door, cut off the lights, and climbed into bed. It's amazing how your bed is such a place of refuge, especially in times of trouble. I didn't know what else to do. My family members were in pain so that I couldn't call them. I didn't want to trouble others with such bad news and hear the "everything will be alright" speech again. I just wanted to bury myself, away from the world and let the numbness take over my body. I felt that was what my grandfather was feeling after receiving the news, and I didn't have the right to try to feel better during his suffering.

A short time later I heard my door creek open, and I felt the glow of the light from the hallway. I had taken the comforter and wrapped it around my body, and after hearing the door open I made the attempt to roll on my side and hide that I was emotionally crushed. I didn't know if I should cry, should yell, should pray, or should go to the land of disbelief on the news, and having Bill walk in at this moment made me feel uncomfortable. I just lay there, and I heard him take soft steps toward my bed. Then he stopped.

I didn't look up. I just lay there, and he just stood there. Gently, Bill sat on the edge of the bed and placed his hand on the center of my back. Then he did the right thing for such a discombobulated moment. He leaned in, and lightly kissed me on the jaw. I immediately sat up and grabbed Bill and began to cry harder than I ever had up to that moment. This began the first stages of my failure.

Death and destruction were my foes for the next six months. I started to not take care of myself because I was emotionally crippled.

On the other side of my family, my Grandmother Cora had been sick for some time. She was in a home, and everyone was doing their best to make her comfortable, but it was only a matter of time. She had dementia, and it was taking away her memories, her day to day functions, and most importantly, it was taking her away from us. She didn't recognize anyone anymore, but my mother religiously went to take care of her. I never went to the hospital to see her due to the fear of death and seeing her in such a state. It is one of my biggest regrets in life. My mother would give updates, and she was coming to grips with the understanding of losing her step-mother, but it didn't make the process easier for anyone. So, grandma was dying on mom's side of the family, grandpa was dying on dad's side of the family, and more heartache was to come.

The holidays came, and we went to Kalamazoo to see my grandfather. When I walked into his home, the first thing I noticed was the walker. You always see older people using walkers, but when it is someone you love, it freaks you out. He was settled in his favorite chair, but the walker was in front, and it bothered me. My grandfather didn't need such a thing! People who are weak need assistance from objects like walkers, and I was in denial that he would need one. I was wrong.

He couldn't move without the walker and had to go to the restroom every 30 minutes. The floors had plastic covering so that he wouldn't slip while trying to walk. There were bars and safety contraptions everywhere for my grandfather, and seeing those items made it official to me that he was terribly sick. He looked the same, but he wasn't inside. He was dying a slow, painful death and I didn't know how to deal with it. So, I began healing the only way I knew how. I ate.

I started eating that day. The band made it so I couldn't pig out, but I ate foods that I didn't need to. I ate heavy foods; I skipped out on vegetables and gave into a cake. I ate the way I use to, and I didn't care about what calories I took in, what starchy foods I ingested, and how full I got. I did this throughout that day, and the next and the next until Christmas came. The holiday spirit wasn't with me. I was so sad and could barely get out of bed some days. I took days off from work and stopped going to lunch with my Spice Girls. I didn't want to face my emotions with all the bad things that were going on.

I didn't know who I could talk to about it. My father was taking the news hard, and my mother was coping as best she could. I didn't want to burden them with my emotional baggage, so I didn't call my parents when I was down. My sister and brother were more emotional people than I, and I was a listening ear to whoever needed to talk or text. Someone had to be everyone's sounding board and had to be strong, and I took on that role for anyone who needed it. The problem was I felt alone, and nothing could fix that feeling.

I was empty, and food would give me a temporary filling after a stressful day at work. My job was making my life even more complicated. When you are the teacher whose job is to get seniors ready to graduate, and juniors to pass state mandated test, the pressure can be mentally and emotionally crippling. So it came to pass for me.

One day another teacher had an issue with me and came banging on my door during my planning. I was on the phone, speaking to my sister and listening to her pain when this teacher came banging on my door like it was a crisis drill. I ignored it the first time, but she continued. I finally had to tell my sister I would call her back in the middle of her crying. This teacher had the nerve to curse at me for not doing something immediately for her, and for a student I had not seen in months. It took every ounce of my strength not to punch that woman in the mouth, scattering her teeth across the hallway floor like confetti on New Year's after the countdown. I was ready, and my fist was balled up to hit her right on the target of her loud, obnoxious mouth. I was ready to walk out on my job and the stress that came with what I do day in and day out. I yelled back, and she proceeded to be rude and say I was out of line for speaking loudly at her. She has no clue how close she came to a dangerous side of me that day. I was depressed, confused, and more importantly, I was doing the best I could. I am usually good at forgiving and forgetting, but I cannot let go of the fact that I could not listen to my sister over a professional's childish behavior. After that "teacher" left, I ate a candy bar. I still hate her to this day.

Grandma Cora died December 30th. I was in bed when my mother called with the news. I was saddened to hear of the loss of my step-grandmother, but I was also strangely relieved for her. She had suffered so much, and she didn't deserve it. She deserved to rest and to be completely at peace after going through years of dementia. My mother's heart was hurt, and I listened to her on the phone. I shared my news with Bill, who quickly asked about my status I calmly told him I was fine. Oddly, I was fine and began to check up on others to make sure everyone was alright.

I coped with my grief by staying home on New Year's Eve, and I stayed in my room and ate more. I drank things I didn't need to drink, and I just laid there. Grandma Cora's funeral was when it hit me that I had lost a family member. It wasn't while we walked in the funeral home as a family. It wasn't when I looked at her body, or the long process of lowering the lid and closing the casket. It was much later.

It hit me at the cemetery.

She was laid to rest in a military cemetery. It was so peaceful once you entered the sacred ground. The entrance, decorated with what seemed to be thousands of flags, sparkled under the sun. It was unusually sunny and warm for a January day. I did not realize the warmth until we finished the ceremony outside near the beautiful water that rippled from a gentle wind. We had to leave her there. We left her there, alone, and that meant the finality of my step-grandmother. I felt something I hadn't in a long time, and my first reaction to the finality all the events was, "I'm hungry."

Now granted, it had been a long day. I hadn't eaten since nine and the time was after three, but I realized that the final step to this day was yet to come. We had to go back to the church and eat to feel better. And that is exactly what I did. I ate the soul food piled on my plate out of dealing with the grief.

The eating became worse with the deteriorating health of my beloved grandfather.

The last time that I saw my grandfather alive was Super bowl Sunday. My brother and I drove to Kalamazoo on our own because we both had to work. The rest of the family had gone ahead of us, and I drove with thousands of thoughts filtering through my brain. My sister and her family had even come in town, and we decided to make this a celebration of my youngest nephew Mikey's birthday.

The whole family would be there, which shows the urgency in the situation to spend time with him while we could.

Cancer had spread quickly. It had gone from his bladder to his hip and throughout his skeletal system. The walker last time scared me, but it was nothing compared to what I was about to see of what was left of my grandfather.

When I walked through the door, all I wanted to see was my grandfather.

The man I saw was not what I remembered of my Paw Paw…

A man who was the first black foreman of GM in Michigan, won countless awards, coached men who entered the NFL, was nothing more than a frail specimen. He was wearing a green neck brace to keep his head up and covered in one of my grandmother's homemade blankets. He was wilting away. He still had on his traditional glasses, perched on his pointy nose, and he still had that bald head that I loved and adored, but that was practically it. He was melting away. I was losing him.

After speaking to him and giving him his traditional pat on the head in greeting, he smiled and said his traditional phrase, "Hey granddaughter." I asked him brief questions and made sure he was enjoying everyone being in the house. He did a small giggle and said he was having a wonderful time. His voice had even changed, and it sounded weary of the world, tired of fighting cancer, but it still had spirit and fight to pacify the family.

I walked to the back room to catch my breath and to suppress my feelings of breaking down. Once I gathered myself together, I went back out and joined the family for the celebration of life. We celebrated the beginning stages of Mikey's life and the end of my Paw Paw's.

We did what we always did; we ate. I did the same. I didn't excuse myself to go and get more health foods; I ate all the fattening foods that family, friends, and the church had to offer. I grazed, I nibbled, and I enjoyed things that I shouldn't have. I made the excuse that I didn't want to offend anyone by leaving, but the truth is I needed comfort.

As my grandfather's health went downward my weight went up. I didn't find joy in many things that I did to get myself on track. I didn't want to work out, I didn't want to go walking, I didn't want to take care of myself, even though I should have.

There were days that I didn't have an appetite, and there were days that I couldn't get full. Bill tried to keep me on track but it was pointless, he couldn't tell me what to do. I was so sad listening to the pain of my parents and watching them run to everyone in the family to be caregivers. There were other family issues, and trying to stay positive was nearly impossible. I was starting to become a failure with my quest to become healthy. Staying successful at losing the weight when your "GB-ed" takes a very careful balance of being healthy physically, mentally, and spiritually, and I was weak in every area.

It was the first day of spring when I last spoke to my grandfather. My parents had left earlier in the week because he was losing the fight, and his body was starting to shut down. I was at work when I received the text from my father to call immediately and say my last words to my grandfather.

It was the fourth hour, my planning period, when I picked up the phone, dialed his number, and said my last words to him.

He couldn't speak back. He had lost the ability to speak. He was struggling to breathe, and could only blink in communication. I said my final words, which I choose not to share and then hung up the phone. I placed my phone on my computer, and just sat behind my desk, feeling numb. Then it happened.

I wept.

I didn't cry; I wept from all the pain crushing my soul. I wept from losing my grandmother, cancer destroying my grandfather, that my job was a thankless one that was becoming more and more unrewarding, that my family was in turmoil. I became angry that God wouldn't give me any answers and was allowing this much pain to hit me at once.

I was sad, confused, and angry. To make matters worse, I still had to teach two more hours, and coach later that day. Since teachers are robots in our society, I had to find a way to collect my emotions and teach a group of seniors who were pretty much centered on one thing, themselves.

I held it together for my fifth hour, but I couldn't when the sixth hour came. One positive about education is every once and awhile you run across a group of kids who truly know you and care about you. I was lucky enough to have two classes like this, my third and sixth hour. To have a class at the end of the day that is bright, friendly, funny and enjoyable is a rare find in teaching, but I had it for this school year.

The bell rang; kids filtered in and took their seats. We were working in the computer lab that day, so my main goal was to hurry up talking and send the kids to the lab. I said only two lines to them when a kid named Courtney stopped me from talking. Courtney was never one shy to speak up, but he had never interrupted me before.

"Ms. Mathews, what's wrong with you?"

A knot quickly formed in my throat, and I couldn't answer. Courtney was so urgent in knowing what was wrong with me that he still hand his hand raised in the air after asking his question. All of my students turned and looked at me, many with confused faces and looks of horror.

Right then and there, my lip began to quiver and I felt my head collapse in my arms resting on my desk. I broke down in front of my class of seniors.

The only phrase I could muster to say was, "Go to the lab, please" and I buried my face in my hands and wept again. Some kids scurried quickly to the lab, horrified by my actions. Three students, including Courtney, refused to leave. Once I raised my head to see them still there, each ran to me and hugged me. I insisted they leave me be, and go work in the lab. I promised I would join them as soon as I could. As the students left, my tutor that hour walked in.

Ms. Sage is one of the kindest people I have ever met. She has a sing-song voice, and the kids love her. She looked at me alarmed, and I briefly stated my problem and I continued to cry. She hopped right into action and said she would be in the lab with the kids, and for me to take my time. "You take all hour if you want, Ms. Mathews, I will do whatever you need me to do."

After Susan left, I kicked my chair over. I punched my desk. After violently attacking my classroom furniture, I wiped my face and looked at myself in the mirror. My face was a disaster, but I had to get back to work. At that moment, I felt something I hadn't before. I felt my band tighten on my stomach. This wasn't like the tightening I had done in the doctor office; it had tightened on its own due to stress. I felt like I couldn't breathe, and stooped over in pain. I panted for air, but I didn't pray. I didn't think that God would hear me. After many moments, I went to finish teaching my class but often had to sit down because I didn't feel well.

The band stayed tight for the rest of the day and throughout the evening. I didn't eat, and I didn't drink. I kept the phone next to my side at all times. I kept looking at the phone, waiting for the death notice of my grandfather, but it never came.

Bill checked on me constantly, and RKB texted to make sure that I hadn't jumped off any buildings. Both knew that I was walking the fine line of sanity with all of the tragedy surrounding me. As much as I appreciate the both of them, it didn't help the pain.

I didn't go to work the next day due to the embarrassment of my breakdown, the lack of sleep, and the tightening of my stomach. I still went to coach because I had to do a required meeting with all the parents that night. Practice went well, and I put on a happy face for all the parents so that they knew that being part of the soccer program was the best choice for their daughter.

Being that fake to people made me even more tired, and I laid down on my loveseat to try to relax. Bill and I were having a conversation over a television program when my phone rang. It was my brother. Paw Paw couldn't fight anymore. He was gone.

I lost my grandfather on March 21,. Hearing the news from my brother was almost stunning to my soul, because he said it so naturally. I replied just as plainly to him and hung up the phone.

I looked at Bill and simply said, "He's gone." Within my haze I heard him say "I'm sorry" but I didn't respond back. I just lay there and I felt nothing until I realized that Bill had slid in next to me on the loveseat and was holding on to me. He told me it was alright to cry, and he wasn't going to move until I did so. I followed his orders. I have no idea how long we stayed like this, but I felt that my world had completely stopped. Nothing made sense anymore.

I felt my band tighten again.

I hit rock bottom after losing my Paw Paw.

I had no motivation toward better health. I started to have a new philosophy on life. I had the surgery to live longer and be healthier, but what was the point when we are all going to die? Did taking the steps toward better health mean anything? My grandfather was a man who was strong, focus, goal-oriented and took his health seriously, but it didn't matter. He wasn't perfect, by no means. He was condescending to some, put work first, didn't play around with us like the typical grandfather, and was a glory hound, but he was mine. In my mind, he was invincible. I learned that he wasn't immortal, and neither was I. At least I could be happy if I had junk food and gave up these crazy ideas of a better life. I saw no purpose, and without purpose, there is no motivation.

I had become a failure.

FOOD REJECTION

If you were to ask me what the worst part of being a banded member, I would tell you that it is the fact that you will have to go through the process of food rejection. It is the most disgusting thing that anyone can go through who had this procedure, but it happens.

Food rejection is a nice way of saying throwing up food that your band doesn't want. Sometimes it happens when you eat too much, sometimes when you eat too fast, and sometimes the band is just being plain stubborn. It can happen after having a band tightening, stomach irritation, or when your band tightens under stress.

Unfortunately, I have gone through this process twice, once with food and once while drinking water. It is nothing like when you get sick with the flu, it is an overwhelming odd feeling that ends with a violent action.

The first food rejection that I had was with food and right after the death of my grandfather. I had not been eating, and the roommate insisted that I make the effort to eat something with substance. He had left for the evening and I had just finished a lame attempt at eating dinner. I could feel my stomach did not approve.

The best way to explain the first stages of food rejection is that it feels like you have a rock settled underneath your diaphragm. I am sure other banded individuals might not agree with this imagery, but I can only speak about my experiences. This rock that is resting in your midsection will not move. As a matter of fact, you realize that there is a problem when your realize you can feel this heaviness not only in the upper parts of your stomach, but also in the center of your back. It aches in the front and the back, and you can't do anything with the pain.

I didn't know how to deal with what was going on. I debated on taking some medicine, and even about drinking some water (in the banded life, you are not supposed to eat and drink at the same time). I decided to lie down and hope that it would pass. It didn't.

My next step was a heavy tongue. My saliva became thicker, and the puffiness in my mouth was making me even more nauseous. I didn't know what to do, and no one was home to help me. The rock in my stomach started to put pressure on my chest and in my throat, and I was rocking in pain.

The beginning stages were terrible, but they were nothing compared to the final moments. I stood up and walked into the restroom. My main objective was to spit out the saliva that kept forming in my mouth. I wasn't choking on the food that was stuck, but I started panting from the discomfort. Suddenly, all hell broke loose.

A food rejection in my experience happens rather quickly and forcefully. I am glad I made it to my toilet. Everything just shoots up out of you, and you can't control the event.

It makes you so tired when you finish. Your head hurts from the force, your jaws will need massaging, and you need to not rush to stand due to the swimming feeling from nausea. I sat on the floor for a couple minutes to get myself together. I eventually dragged myself back into my room and laid back on my bed.

The stress had gotten the best of me, and I saw this as a sign that I was struggling to get myself back on track. If I didn't eat, I was not taking care of myself. If I did eat, I might get sick. I didn't know what to do.

Like my dinner, I was stuck.

FIVE YEARS TO THE DAY

Things had changed so much.

On the anniversary of my surgery, I rose early in the morning, thinking of the changes I had made for myself. I had one thing in mind when I rose that morning. Progress. How far had I progressed?

After tossing back the soccer comfort blanket that Damiekco had given me during the season, I placed my feet on the ground, rose from my mattress, and headed down the main hallway. The weather was comfortable, but there was a slight chill throughout the house. The temperature was nice, but a shiver went down my back as I reached the hallway storage door. It was a place that we kept recycling, old clothing, and house hold cleaning supplies. But there was something special in this place. Something that had been put on the highest shelf, collecting dust for the past five years. It was so tucked away that I had to raise on the tips of my toes to reach it. The item escaped my fingers and hit the brown carpet with a thud, and I took a minute to stare at a part of my past.

My biggest pair of pants.

These were my "tight" jeans when I made the decision to have surgery. My jeans that were used on dress down Fridays at work with my students, or when I stepped out on a night on the town with friends. They were the most reliable item in my closet before surgery. Bill and I had put them there once they had become baggy, and we vowed not to touch them until the time was right. All my other clothes from the past were donated to different charities or tossed out with gusto to be picked up on trash day. I didn't want any of those clothes to remain in my house. They had to leave my presence. These jeans were the only things that I saved. I had to know if I had changed. The time was to be on this day.

I scooped up my pile of denim and rushed to Bill's room. He was half-awake but visually annoyed that I barged into his room. He blinked out the sleepiness in his eyes and rolled over to his side. I stood in the doorway of his room, begging for him to wake up.

"I need you to come up front. It's important. And take my phone. I need you to take a picture."

There was a grunt thrown in my direction and a rolling of the eyes. I couldn't blame him for being irritated. It was his summer break, and he deserved to sleep. But, that didn't change the urgency of the situation. I had training that morning with MSU and had to head out in a short time. I am aware that bothering this man was childish, but, I wanted him to be the person to share this moment with me. He was the first that I shared with in the idea of having surgery, and he would be the first to either cheer with me or scoop me off the ground from crying.

"Biiiiiiilllllllllllll! Please get up. It's a big day! Its anniversary day and I need you! Get up! Get up! Get up!"

After a few moments of me groveling, he finally sat up. There were curse words being mumbled under his breath as he headed up front. He then crashed on the couch, still hazy from the dreams the night before. I tossed him my phone.

"It's been five years, friend."

"I know." Bill rubbed his eyes and yawned. "I can't believe I survived you for that long."

I smack my lips and cut my eyes in his direction. I unfolded the wrinkled pants, and I held them out in the sunlight coming through the window.

I wore a black spandex fitness top and leggings to start the day. I'm held up the pants, studying the waistband. I fit these. I remember wearing these pants like it was yesterday. Was it five years ago when I wore these? Time seem to move so fast. Bill's comment made me turn my head in his direction, and away from the jeans.

"Go put them on and come back out. I'll wait here. Go on. You woke me up for this, so get yourself ready."

Once again, I found myself standing in front of the bathroom mirror. I wasn't looking at myself, begging for change. I was standing there to measure progress. This time, I didn't want to have a tear run down my cheek, begging myself to find a way to live longer and happier. I was there to see change.

I slipped the jeans over my leggings. At first, I didn't realize a shift in weight. I did the zipper and buttoned up the waist. Then, I just stood there and stared. I didn't need to do the zipper nor do up the button. I could have just slipped them on fastened. They could have slipped them on like the leggings that I wore too. I didn't need to do the accessories on the jeans. Since when could I do that with my previously tight jeans? I couldn't believe it.

I ran out the bathroom to the couch. Bill was now awake and surfing the net on his phone. He glanced up over his glasses and smiled. I stood there, holding my pants up with both hands, staring in amazement at the changes. This much weight loss couldn't have happened in five years. It just couldn't have! I was in disbelief.

"Well, I guess you have your answer on if you lost weight. I knew you had. And deep down, you knew you had too. Just seeing how much you lost... It's pretty amazing."

I agreed with him. "Amazing" was the right word. The material was gathered in my palms, and a smile was spread across my face. I had changed. A lot.

"Turn so we can do one of those classic pictures people do when they lose weight. Pull the front of the band of your pants out. Let's see how much it is."

I followed Bill's instructions and turned sideways. After gathering up my pants so that they were properly at my waist line, I stretched the material out in front of me. The band was inches from my body. There was the just space between the jeans and I. Five years ago that space was filled with me. Now, there was just an orbit surrounding me. My bottom lip started to shake, but I refused to cry. Not now. I had already shed so many tears in this process. All I wanted to do was smile.

"Look here and smile. You deserve to grin after this, Jes. Good job."

Bill took quick shots with my camera; I quickly changed my clothing for MSU training, and I rushed out the door. I took the jeans with me. I wanted opinions on what to do with the jeans when the day was complete. Maybe my friends could help me figure out what to do with them.

There was a side of me that wanted the damn things to suffer. Others agreed. One new friend, Melanie, understood what I was feeling. She told me to burn them. Turn them into ashes and to throw them into the air like party time confetti. I think she understood my feeling better than anyone else. While others were coming up with sweet ways to deal with the pants, she wanted me to be violent with them.

An opinion came from the corner of the Media Center. "Jes, maybe make them into a bag."

"Wait, what about saving them for another five years and measuring again?"

Another woman chimed in. "No, make them a blanket. That way you could keep the memories of the past you."

But another plus size diva, Jessica, wasn't having all that cheerfulness with the jeans. She was feverishly shaking her head at each one of the ideas.

"Jessyca, destroy them. The old you is gone, and so the jeans need to go. Cut them up. Put them somewhere where they will never hurt you again. You don't want them around anymore. They have served their purpose and they need to get gone from you. Do it, girl."

Jessica had a point. I didn't want them around anymore. Keeping them could destroy what hard work I had done. I tapped my toe furiously on the old school library carpet. I always tap my foot when I am deep in thought.

"I do have one suggestion in keeping the memory of them if you feel you need motivation."

Jessica's statement demanded my attention. I turned and listened only to her, as others continued to talk about the work that we were doing or what to do with jeans.

"Cut out the size. It's the only thing that you need to keep. Save that number and remember that you will never be that number ever again. That number does not represent you but remember that number. Cut it out, put it somewhere, and when you find it from time to time, you will smile."

She was right. That was the only thing that I needed to keep. That number pressed into the fabric was my number a short time ago. I was so obese then that my jean size was 26. I was 318 pounds when I wore those pants. 318. No longer was I the number 26 or 318. Things had changed. I had changed. I was ready to move on.

Goodbye, size 26.

Goodbye, 318.

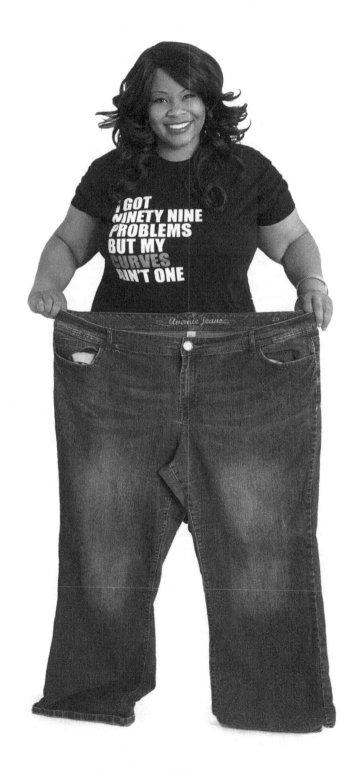

ACKNOWLEDGEMENTS

Mom & Dad: You instilled a drive within me to be a good person and to follow my heart. Without your hard work and guidance, I would be nothing. You are the best and I love you.

Bill: Thank you for putting up with my hungry days, my emotional mood swings in this process, and keeping me focused. I adore you, always.

My Bariatric Team: You saved my life. I am forever grateful. Each of you deserve my gratitude, especially Dr. Farhan and Nurse Nancy.

RKB: To my biggest encourager over the years. To steal your quote in our friendship, "Thank you for being you." I heart you.

Grandma Cora: I'm a diva today because you can't be here to set the standard, grandma. I miss your smile.

Paw Paw: I fell after you left, but I got up swinging. That's what a Mathews is meant to do. Please brag about me in heaven.

Family, friends, and students: Thank you for your kind words and positive thoughts. You helped me to make it through each day, especially Nurse Angi and my Christobal.

People who go doubted me: Please continue to do so. It just drives me to be a better person.

Photographer Alex, Editor Earlexus, and Beta Susan: Thank you for making this book come to life. Blessings to all of you and I am forever grateful.

Damiekco: You were the final piece to finishing the first stage of the journey. Don't forget that, "I got you too" always. I blame you, so very much.

Finally, and most importantly, thank you *Lord* for my strength, stubbornness, and tunnel vision on life. I am nothing without you. I am blessed beyond measure.

ABOUT THE AUTHOR

Jessyca Mathews is an English teacher in Flint, Michigan. She is a graduate of *Marygrove College* in Detroit, Michigan, with a degree in Master in the Art of Teaching. She also attended the *University of Michigan-Flint* to receive her English Degree with a specialization in Secondary Education and is a fellow of the *National Writing Project* through her work with the *Red Cedar Writing Project* at *Michigan State University*. After having the strength to complete her gastric banding surgery in 2011, she has enjoyed many successes and awards in writing and community service.

Her first published book, *Simply: A Collection of Poetry* is an award-winning piece from a national contest with MANA. She has begun doing motivational speeches and poetry readings at different events in the state of Michigan. She continues to write about her experiences and is working on publishing an additional poetry collection and memoir.

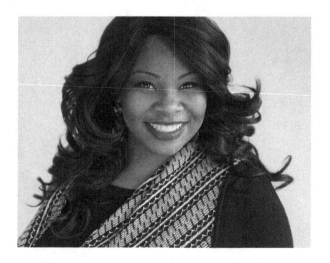

Printed in the United States
By Bookmasters